Contents

KT-363-242

Tables

Figures

Moving up with diabetes

The transition from paediatric to adult care

Jessica Datta

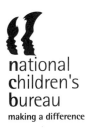

national
children's
bureau

making a difference

The National Children's Bureau promotes the interests and well-being of all children and young people across every aspect of their lives. NCB advocates the participation of children and young people in all matters affecting them. NCB challenges disadvantage in childhood.

NCB achieves its mission by
- ensuring the views of children and young people are listened to and taken into account at all times
- playing an active role in policy development and advocacy
- undertaking high quality research and work from an evidence based perspective
- promoting multidisciplinary, cross-agency partnerships
- identifying, developing and promoting good practice
- disseminating information to professionals, policy makers, parents and children and young people

NCB has adopted and works within the UN Convention on the Rights of the Child.

Cover:
Molecular model of the insulin molecule, ribbon representation.
T. Blundell and N. Campillo/Wellcome Photo Library.

Published by the National Children's Bureau, Registered Charity number 258825. 8 Wakley Street, London EC1V 7QE. Tel: 020 7843 6000. Website: www.ncb.org.uk

© National Children's Bureau, 2003
Published 2003

ISBN 1 900990 94 6

British Library Cataloguing in Publication Data
A catalogue record for this book is available from the British Library

Acknowledgements

First, I would like to thank the young people who generously contributed their time and shared their experiences, views and ideas for this project. Altogether 225 young people participated including those who were interviewed, those who filled in a questionnaire, those who contacted us through the internet and those who attended a consultation day on diabetes and the internet.

Many thanks too to the diabetes specialist nurses and doctors at the six hospitals included in the study who identified the samples of young people, distributed letters on our behalf and collected background information on the services they provide. Thanks to all the health care staff who made themselves available, despite busy schedules, to be interviewed for the study and shared their views on and their aspirations for the care of young people with diabetes.

Thanks are also due to the members of the project's advisory group who offered their expertise, attended meetings and gave helpful advice. They are Wendy Beecher, Carol Carson, David Dunger, Ross Grindley, Graham Hood, Ian Jefferson, Richard Olsen, Andrew Pasterfield, Dominic Patterson, Chas Skinner and Alexandra Smith. Special thanks go to Carol Carson, who attended the Diabetes Internet Day and brought four young people from Edinburgh with her, and to Dominic Patterson, who allowed us to post a questionnaire on his website Diabetes Explained (www.diabetes-explained.co.uk). Thanks also to Diabetes UK, a charity working for people with diabetes, whose staff provided invaluable assistance.

Thanks too to Nicola Madge who developed the research proposal and supervised the project. Carol Carson and Richard Olsen read the report in draft and made useful comments on the text.

The study could not have been carried out without the help of the field workers who interviewed many of the participants. Thanks to Tracy Dickinson, Sophie Sarre and Anne Scott. Thanks also to colleagues at Children In Scotland for supporting the project and especially to Anne-Marie Dorian and Evelyn McGregor who interviewed both young people and hospital staff.

I would also like to thank Professor Clare Bradley of the Psychology Department at Royal Holloway, University of London, who allowed us to use the ADDQoL-Teen, the quality of life measure for young people with diabetes. Thanks also to Professor Bradley and Dr Carolyn McMillan for the analysis of the quality of life data.

Thanks for administrative support, particularly the transcription of interviews, to Ruth Ramanan and Kate Walters and to Claire Clayton and her team.

The project was generously supported by the Community Fund.

Jessica Datta
May 2003

1. Introduction

The incidence and prevalence of diabetes in children and young people is increasing in Britain (SIGN 2001). Although most young people can effectively manage living with diabetes, there is evidence that some face a worse outcome than may be necessary. Concern has been voiced about the consistency of standards of care for people with diabetes and, in particular, about the arrangements for the transfer from paediatric to adult care for young people. Diabetes services that are not tailored to the needs of adolescents may be rejected by them and cause them not to seek medical help when necessary.

There are no national standards for the transfer of young people with diabetes from paediatric to adult services determining, for example, the age at which young people make the move to adult care. Although good practice guidelines produced by Diabetes UK (BDA 1995), SIGN (2001) and ISPAD (2000) make a number of recommendations about services for young people and how transition should be managed, in practice there are many different arrangements which can depend on a number of local factors. Caseload size, available resources, geographical location, relationships, the level of cooperation between the paediatric and adult services and local philosophies may all play a part in how transition is managed in a particular hospital.

Little detailed information is available about these different arrangements and one of the aims of this study is to describe different models of clinic practice for young people with diabetes, focusing particularly on procedures surrounding transfer from paediatric to adult services. The study also explores the views of both young people and health care professionals on diabetes services and examines young people's attendance and non-attendance at diabetes clinics, quality of life and the effect of diabetes, the support available from friends and family and at school, and young people's information needs.

Diabetes and adolescence

Concern has been raised about young people with diabetes for a number of
reasons. These include both their short- and long-term health, their ability to
maintain quality of life in the adolescent years and their psychological
functioning. Research has shown that adolescence is a time when glycaemic
control can be poor, when diabetic emergencies are more common than in
other age groups, and when signs of medical complications associated with
diabetes may be detected. There have been improvements in young people's
diabetes control but it is still not optimal and there is a high incidence of
complications reported in young adults (Betts *et al.* 2002). Although
complications are unusual among children, poor glycaemic control in
adolescence coupled with long duration of the condition are indicators of
increased risk of complications. There is particular concern about the onset of
complications for young people who were diagnosed with diabetes in early
childhood and who have therefore been living with the condition for a number
of years. Mortality rates in children and young people with diabetes are higher
than in the general population (Edge, *et al.* 1999).

The Diabetes Control and Complications Trial (DCCT 1993) showed that
lowering blood glucose concentration slows or prevents the development of
diabetic complications such as retinopathy and neuropathy. The principal aim
of diabetes management therefore is to maintain optimal blood glucose control
which can only be achieved by the commitment of the person living with
diabetes with advice and support from medical staff. There is evidence that
young people may not seek medical care at the point at which they move from
paediatric to adult care or in the following years (Kipps *et al.* 2002). Guidelines
on the care of adolescents have made recommendations for how services can
make the best provision for this age group and, in the last few years, many
hospital diabetes teams have adapted their services to accommodate young
people in order to ensure they have access to appropriate care.

It seems that there are both physiological and social reasons why glycaemic
control can deteriorate in the adolescent years. The National Paediatric
Diabetes Audit (Smith 2001) found mean levels of HbA1c (glycated
haemoglobin or blood glucose) went up as children's age increased, especially
with the onset of puberty. Puberty and growth may have an effect on the ability
of young people to maintain optimal glycaemic control. Insulin sensitivity is at
its lowest during mid-adolescence and is related to circulating growth hormone
concentrations (Acerini *et al.* 2000). The increase in growth hormone and

accompanying physiological insulin resistance in this period means adolescents with diabetes are likely to have greater insulin requirements and these may need to be adjusted regularly. The National Paediatric Diabetes Audit (Smith 2001) found that HbA1c in this age group also increased with duration of diabetes. This could also be an effect of puberty but may be caused by poorer compliance with treatment.

Adolescence is a time when young people become increasingly responsible and independent, experiment with new behaviours, take risks with their health and forge 'grown up' identities. Diabetes may interfere with new found freedoms and friendships, and pressure to conform with peers and not appear 'different' may be strong. School work is more demanding during this period and stress associated with exams may also have an effect on diabetes control. Increased independence and changes in lifestyle in teenagers may make them less willing to adhere closely to a tight regimen of insulin injections, diet and exercise. The increase in the incidence of diabetes in very young children means that there will be a growing number of adolescents who have been living with diabetes for ten or more years (Gardner *et al.* 1997).

Some young people with diabetes may experience psychological and social difficulties in adolescence which have serious consequences for short- and long-term health. Diabetes mismanagement is not unusual in adolescents and is more prevalent as they grow older (Wiessberg-Benchell *et al.* 1995). Research has found poorer HbA1c levels in young women than in young men (La Greca *et al.* 1995a, Bryden *et al.* 1999) and more episodes of diabetic ketoacidosis (DKA) and hospitalisations related to diabetes (Brink 1997). Omission or under-use of insulin in order to lose weight is associated with episodes of DKA and poor glycaemic control and is more commonly associated with young women (Peveler *et al.* 1992, Gill 1993, Morris *et al.* 1997, Bryden *et al.* 1999, Meltzer *et al.* 2001, Neumark-Sztainer *et al.* 2002, Nissim *et al.* 2002). Others allow their blood glucose levels to run higher than optimal in order to avoid episodes of hypoglycaemia. Research carried out in Canada (Jones *et al.* 2000) found the proportion of young women aged between 12 and 19 with type 1 diabetes displaying eating disorders was almost twice as high as in a sample without diabetes. The study also found that young women with diabetes who suffered from eating disorders had poorer glycaemic control than those who did not. There is also evidence that behavioural problems in the teenage years are related to higher mean HbA1c levels in young adulthood and, therefore, to the higher risks of medical complications associated with increased blood glucose levels (Bryden *et al.* 2001). In contrast, an international study found that young people who had better glycaemic control reported better quality of life than those with higher blood glucose levels (Hoey *et al.* 2001).

Diabetes services for young people

Standard 5 of the National Service Framework for Diabetes (DH 2001) states:

> All children and young people with diabetes will receive
> consistently high-quality care and they, with their families
> and others involved in their day-to-day care, will be
> supported to optimise the control of their blood glucose and
> their physical, psychological, intellectual, educational and
> social development.

The Standard has not yet been fully implemented and there is evidence that standards of care for people with diabetes are not consistent across England and Wales and that the pressure on services will increase as patient numbers rise (Audit Commission 2000). Although there is a rise in the number of children and young people diagnosed with type 1 diabetes, the greatest increase is in the incidence of type 2 in the older population which accounts for 85 to 90 per cent of cases. This rise in type 2 diabetes is associated with an aging population, obesity and a sedentary lifestyle and ethnic minority communities who are more likely to be affected. Surveys carried out over a number of years on behalf of Diabetes UK (Jefferson *et al.* 2003) also raised concerns that there are still hospitals where children with diabetes do not receive the specialised paediatric care recommended by guidelines and that the full range of expert support staff is not always available although the picture is steadily improving. The surveys showed, for example, that the provision of dietetic advice and of psychological support is lacking in many clinics. This disparity between services is of great concern in terms of both equity and outcome. International studies of diabetes clinics serving children and young people have shown a great variation in levels of glycaemic control between centres indicating that the quality of services can affect outcomes. The explanation for such variations seems to be associated with organisational details of care such as the time allocated to individual children and their families and the approach of professionals as well as psychological and cultural factors (Betts and Swift 2003). The National Paediatric Diabetes Audit also found significant differences in HbA1c results between diabetes services for children in Britain. However, it is difficult to compare results because there is no national standard for measuring glucose in blood and it is therefore not possible to say whether like is being compared with like. Paediatricians have called for 'a uniform, equitable and first class paediatric service throughout the UK' (Betts *et al.* 2002) and for increased collaboration with adult colleagues to enable a successful transition to an adult service which meets the needs of young people, encourages their attendance and improves both their diabetes control and quality of life. The National Service Framework for Diabetes: Delivery Strategy (DH 2003) includes guidance on the establishment of effective registers for all people with diabetes which would be helpful both for follow-up of individuals and also for epidemiological studies of the incidence and prevalence of type 1 diabetes.

Timing and location of clinics, the quality of patient/staff relationships and continuity of care are all factors in providing appropriate services. Failure to attend appointments which results in a lack of monitoring of glycaemic control may have devastating effects on individual young people but also has an impact on health service budgets. Preventive services which monitor control on a regular basis may be considered expensive but if they result in 'healthier patients, less complications, reduced intervention and less expensive treatments' (Carson 2000), they can be cost effective in the long run. The cost of diabetes is a heavy and increasing burden on health service budgets. According to the Audit Commission (2000), diabetes services form 5 per cent of National Health Service expenditure costing over £2 billion per year. The bulk of this is accounted for by the majority who have type 2 diabetes. The added expense of welfare benefits for those with diabetes related disability add to the public cost of poorly controlled diabetes.

Standard 3 of the National Service Framework for Diabetes (DH 2001) states that:

> all children, young people and adults with diabetes will
> receive a service which encourages partnership in decision-
> making, supports them in managing their diabetes and helps
> them to adopt and maintain a healthy lifestyle.

Increasingly users of health services of all ages are being recognised as central participants in the care team and this is particularly the case for people with chronic conditions like diabetes for whom self-care is crucial to maintaining good health. The person with diabetes lives with the condition every day and is in a position to adapt care to fit the particular needs and circumstances of daily life because 'neither the disease not its consequences are static' (Holman and

Lorig 2000). Cradock (1998), for example, argues that 'when people develop diabetes, they, and only they, become the significant health care provider'. Young people need the support and advice of professionals to gradually develop and understand this role when it is appropriate for them and when they are able and willing to take it on.

Transition to adult care

Young people with diabetes are a group who face increased risks to their long-term health and who may not have access to the most appropriate medical care. The point at which young people move from paediatric to adult care may be critical because it is at this stage that they are increasingly likely to be making their own decisions about diabetes care with less support from their parents. 'Transition in health care is only one part of the wider evolution from dependent child to independent adult' (David 2001) and this evolution is 'physiological, hormonal, psychological and environmental' (Eiser 1996). Services for this age group should take account of all these factors and of the interplay between them. Young people's own lives will also be changing. Some will leave home to go to university and others may be starting their first job. If the transition to adult care is not well managed, young people may stay away from clinic appointments. Service providers should consider the flexibility of the appointment system, the timing of clinics, the approach of staff and the availability and quality of educational resources.

Although there are currently no national standards for the transfer of young people with diabetes from paediatric to adult services, the importance of transition to adult care has been acknowledged by the Department of Health (2001) in the National Service Framework for Diabetes. Standard 6 states:

> All young people with diabetes will experience a smooth transition of care from paediatric diabetes services to adult diabetes services, whether hospital or community-based, either directly or via a young people's clinic. The transition will be organised in partnership with each individual and at an age appropriate to and agreed with them.

Many diabetes services have responded to concerns about young people with diabetes by developing special clinics for this age group although others may continue to transfer patients in 'a haphazard and idiosyncratic fashion' (Viner 1999). These clinics can be jointly run between paediatric and adult services ensuring continuity of care for young people as they 'move up' to adult care. In some hospitals there are also clinics for young adults who have recently moved to adult care or who may have been diagnosed in early adulthood. However, there are no standardised arrangements for this transfer of care. Depending on caseload size, local philosophies and available resources, the age of transfer can differ as can the length of time young people are able to attend 'transition' (or 'adolescent' or 'teenage') clinics. In some clinics, both doctors consult with a young person (with or without a parent present) together while in others young people alternate consultations between a paediatrician and an adult physician.

Despite recent service developments, Russell Viner considers that 'arranging efficient and caring transfer for adolescents from paediatric to adult care is one of the great challenges facing paediatrics – and indeed the health services – in the coming century' (Viner 1999). Young people moving to adult care come face to face with the differing paradigms of paediatric and adult medicine. The former tends to be family centred and focused on development while the latter recognises patient autonomy and issues such as employment but neglects growth, development and family circumstances. Viner acknowledges that the transition to adult care is one of many transitions young people are facing in their teenage years and sees it not as 'an administrative event' but as 'a guided educational and therapeutic process'. The American Society for Adolescent Medicine's definition of transition also describes it as a process rather than a one-off event calling it 'the purposeful, planned movement of adolescents and young adults with chronic physical and medical conditions from child-centred to adult-oriented health care systems' (Blum *et al.* 1993). Obstacles to successful transition can include poorly organised administrative systems, paediatricians who may be reluctant to 'let go' of patients they may have known since babyhood, adolescents and their families who may be unwilling to leave a trusted service and adult physicians whose large caseloads of older patients may leave them little time for young patients.

Viner (1999) suggests that there are key elements for an effective transition programme. These elements include:

- a target age for transfer (with the possibility of flexibility depending on each individual's level of development, health status and circumstances);
- a period before transfer when young people are offered education which prepares them for the increased personal responsibility for their own care expected by adult services and teaches them the skills to make best use of those services;

- a coordinated transfer process which would include providing details of what a young person can expect from adult care, the opportunity to meet staff in the adult service and the provision of a young adult clinic;
- an interested and capable adult service;
- administrative support for the transfer;
- the involvement of primary care staff who may provide the only medical continuity for young people and their families.

Young people with diabetes are identified as a special group who should continue to be looked after by specialist teams into adulthood (ISPAD 2000, SIGN 2001). This inevitably means that they should be registered with a secondary care service although, if they are unwilling to attend a specialist clinic, it is important that they maintain contact with primary care services.

The timing of transfer to adult care is not standardised across services. Some paediatric clinics stop seeing young people when they are 15 or 16 or even younger while others continue to invite young people to a jointly run transition clinic until they are in their early twenties. These differences are determined by both the availability of resources (such as consultant time and clinic space), local priorities and the circumstances in which the service was developed. Transfer to adult care is linked to young people taking increasing responsibility for their own self-care with less input from parents. Some may have the maturity to begin to take on this responsibility in their early teens when they have made the transition to secondary school while others may not be ready for some years. Guidelines suggest that the timing of transfer should take into account 'a young person's stage of physical development, emotional maturity and stated requirements' (BDA 1995).

However, one of the difficulties for clinic staff is deciding when the time is optimal for most young people to make the transition to a jointly run clinic or, if that is not available, to adult care. At 16 young people are facing public exams and may then be moving to a further education college or starting work. At 17 and 18 they are likely to be sitting more exams. At 18 many will be leaving home to go to university and may face another transition if they decide to attend a diabetes clinic in a new town during term time. Although some flexibility should be possible, a target age is probably best so that young people can be prepared for the move and will transfer as part of a cohort who may already know each other from having attended the same paediatric clinic. Services which have smaller caseloads may have the opportunity to be more flexible than large city services where the pressure of patient numbers is greater. Kipps *et al.*

(2002) found that patients who had transferred to adult care at a younger age were more likely to express satisfaction with the transfer process. However, researchers were wary of concluding that earlier transfer was preferable to later as other factors may have been present in determining opinions.

The extent to which young people are educated about self-care and how to make the most of consultations is variable. The establishment of adolescent clinics in many hospitals which are jointly run by paediatric and adult staff may serve Viner's dual aims of providing a well managed transition process and of easing young people into adult services with the confidence to make the most of what they find there. The opportunity for young people to meet members of the adult team (while maintaining contact with paediatric staff) provided by jointly run clinics is also an opportunity for adult staff who may learn from their paediatric colleagues and take an interest in the care of young people. They will also have the chance to meet and get to know young patients before they move to adult care.

Clearly administrative support for the smooth transfer to adult care is important if patients are not to be lost to follow-up. If young people are leaving home to go to university it may be difficult to maintain contact with them even though they may decide to continue to use diabetes care in their home town. As young people leave paediatric services, they need to be aware of what services are available for them to move on to and be given the opportunity to discuss alternatives, if available, so that the likelihood of future non-attendance at clinic appointments is minimised. Young people who are well prepared and therefore confident about the options for their care are more likely to make informed choices about what is best for them.

The transition process is not the end of the story. A worrying number of young people fail to attend clinic appointments in the years after they transfer to adult care (Kipps *et al.* 2002). Adult services need the staff and resources to ensure that young adults are offered acceptable and accessible services in order to encourage them to continue to attend clinic appointments and comply with treatment.

The study

Little detailed information is available about the different transition arrangements offered by hospitals and one of the aims of this study is to describe different models of clinic practice for young people with diabetes, focusing particularly on procedures surrounding transfer from paediatric to adult services. The study examined services available in six areas in Britain which present both common and disparate elements. They all provide services for children and young people with diabetes but their transition arrangements differ. These services are described in Chapter 3.

Another central aim of the study was to elicit the views of young people with diabetes themselves. Young people were asked about their experiences of attending clinic appointments, their views on transferring to adult care, their information needs and their ideas for improving services. Young people's non-attendance at clinic appointments and the failure of some to keep in contact with medical services were also explored. In total, 225 young people and over 30 health care professionals participated in the study.

2.   About diabetes

There are two main types of diabetes – or diabetes mellitus to give it its full name. Children and young people are most likely to have type 1 which means they are dependent on insulin.

Type 1 (or insulin dependent) diabetes

Type 1 diabetes usually occurs in childhood, adolescence or young adulthood and is the third most common chronic condition in children after asthma and cerebral palsy (Audit Commission 2000). Over the last twenty years, the incidence of diabetes in young people has been rising. One regional study, for example, found an annual increase in incidence of 4 per cent per year in children under 15 between 1985 and 1995. Most of this was due to a rise of 11 per cent a year in children under five years in whom incidence doubled over the decade (Gardner *et al.* 1997). Other local studies have also found that childhood diabetes is increasing (Rangasami *et al.* 1997, Feltbower *et al.* 2000). Analysis of the General Practice Research Database (Newnham *et al.* 2002) showed that between 1994 and 1998 the prevalence of insulin treated diabetes increased by 23 per cent. This figure includes young adults with type 1 diabetes and those with type 2 who are insulin dependent and not simply children and adolescents with diabetes. It shows, however, the large advance in the number of people living with diabetes.

Data from the 1980s and 1990s showed the incidence of children under 15 with type 1 diabetes was around 14 per 100,000 per year but more recent data suggests this has now risen to 20 cases per 100,000 population. There are at least 20,000 children and young people with diabetes in the UK and, in Scotland, the annual incidence is 25 per 100,000 (Rangasami *et al.* 1997). The causes for this increase are not clear and the lack of a national database makes it impossible to report accurate figures for the UK.

The incidence of type 1 diabetes varies across European countries. Data from children diagnosed between 1989 and 1990, for example, show wide ranging incidence rates of 4.6 per 100,000 in northern Greece and 42.9 per 100,000 in two regions of Finland (Green *et al.* 1992). It is believed that a complex interaction between genetic and environmental factors is responsible for this variation.

Why does type 1 diabetes occur?

It is not known why type 1 diabetes occurs although epidemiological studies have identified a number of possible risk factors. Mothers' diet in late pregnancy (Shiell *et al.* 2000), mothers' pre-eclampsia in pregnancy (Jones *et al.* 1998), birth weight (Stene *et al.* 2001), early exposure to cow's milk proteins (Akerblom *et al.* 2002), children's rate of growth in their early years (Bruining 2000), social mixing in infancy and the related exposure to infection (McKinney 2000, Parslow *et al.* 2001) and the quality of drinking water (Stene *et al.* 2002) have all been linked with the likelihood of a child or young person developing diabetes but no conclusions have been drawn about what precisely triggers the condition. There may be a genetic predisposition and/or environmental causes which prompt the onset of diabetes although, in most cases, there does not seem to be a known genetic link. Only about a quarter of sufferers have a close family member who also has type 1 diabetes and children are three times more likely to develop diabetes if their father has it rather than their mother (Gale and Gillespie 2001). It is thought that diabetes develops when the body's autoimmune system reacts abnormally to the beta cells in the pancreas. This may be prompted by a virus or other infection although why some people react in this way while others do not is not yet understood.

What happens when you get type 1 diabetes?

Type 1 diabetes is an autoimmune disease in which antibodies destroy the beta cells in the pancreas that produce insulin. Insulin is a hormone which normally controls the amount of glucose in the blood. Glucose is taken into the body from the food that we eat and, after absorption of what has been eaten, the glucose level in the blood rises and insulin is released into the blood. When the glucose level falls, if we take any physical exercise for example, the insulin level also falls. Insulin is important because it regulates the level of glucose in the blood, preventing it from rising too high or falling too low.

Type 1 diabetes begins when the beta cells are so badly damaged that they are unable to make insulin. As the cells are gradually destroyed the warning signs of diabetes appear. Insulin levels are low and therefore glucose cannot enter the cells to act as fuel and instead passes into the urine and is wasted. This process causes ketones and fat to build up in the blood making the blood sugar rise and the blood become more acidic. Sufferers can quite suddenly develop acute symptoms – excessive thirst, frequent urination, extreme tiredness and weight loss – and, in a previously healthy young person, a diagnosis of diabetes should not be difficult to make. If not diagnosed quickly, symptoms may become so serious that emergency hospital admission is necessary. If diabetes is untreated, the person can become dangerously ill with diabetic ketoacidosis (DKA) which can cause multiple system failure and death.

Treating diabetes

Because the body can no longer produce insulin, people with type 1 diabetes need to replace it by injecting insulin regularly. This injected insulin is either derived from animals or is genetically engineered 'human' insulin. Insulin is a protein and therefore cannot be swallowed because enzymes would break it down in the digestive tract. At present, there is no cure for diabetes so sufferers need to inject insulin for the rest of their lives. Like the rest of the population, people with diabetes are encouraged to eat a healthy, balanced diet, take regular exercise and not to smoke.

The first aim of diabetes management is to control blood glucose levels by balancing insulin with food intake and exercise. Ideally injections of insulin should replicate the way the pancreas would release it normally. A normal blood glucose level would be between 4 and 7 millilitres of glucose per litre of blood. A reading under 4 millilitres could cause hypoglycaemia and over 9 millilitres could cause hyperglycaemia.

Although people with diabetes risk developing a number of medical complications, the Diabetes Control and Complications Trial (DCCT 1993) provided evidence that improved diabetes control from diagnosis can reduce the incidence and delay the progression of complications.

Hypoglycaemia

People with well-controlled diabetes can suffer occasional hypoglycaemic reactions or 'hypos' when the blood glucose level drops low. In fact, the better a person's glycaemic control, the more likely they are to experience hypos. Hypo symptoms can include feeling shaky or confused, sweating or going pale. These are the effects of adrenalin being released which acts to move glucose out of body tissues that can survive without it into organs, such as the brain, that need it immediately. Mild hypos can be treated by eating a sweet and fast-acting carbohydrate contained in glucose tablets or sugary drinks followed by more substantial food such as a sandwich or a bowl of cereal which provides a longer-acting carbohydrate. In most cases, people with diabetes can treat the symptoms themselves but sometimes hypoglycaemia can be unexpected or severe and intervention by another person will be necessary.

Hyperglycaemia and diabetic ketoacidosis

Hyperglycaemia occurs if the level of glucose in the blood is too high and is caused when the body does not have enough insulin or cannot use the insulin it does have to convert glucose into energy. When patients are first diagnosed with diabetes they are likely to have symptoms of hyperglycaemia – extreme thirst, a dry mouth and a need to urinate often.

For people with type 1 diabetes, untreated hyperglycaemia may lead to diabetic ketoacidosis (DKA). This begins slowly and builds up over a period when diabetes is out of control and blood glucose levels are too high. Ketones accumulate in the blood and can become toxic. DKA may occur because of illness or under-dosing of insulin but the primary reason is not taking sufficient insulin. Symptoms include nausea and vomiting, stomach pain and rapid breathing, dry skin and a dry mouth, breath that smells of acetone, a weak and rapid pulse and high blood sugar. It must be treated immediately by giving fluids and insulin as ketoacidosis can lead to coma, cerebral oedema and even death. It is the most common cause of death in young people with diabetes (Edge *et al.* 1999).

Medical complications of diabetes

If, over a period of time, blood glucose levels continue to be higher than normal, both blood vessels and nerves can be affected. Microvascular complications, caused by impairment to the small blood vessels, can have an effect on the healing of wounds, cause haemorrhages in the eyes, which impair vision, poor circulation and ulcers, and damage kidneys. Uncontrolled diabetes also affects the larger blood vessels causing macrovascular complications and, with high blood pressure, contributes to cardiovascular disease (damage to the heart and blood circulation). Diabetes-related complications can include renal and cardiac disease, neuropathy (nerve damage) and may lead to visual impairment and limb amputation. Although complications are rare in children, poorly controlled diabetes can lead to poor physical development especially in terms of growth (Bateman 1990).

Women with diabetes are encouraged to be extra vigilant with their glycaemic control before conceiving and during pregnancy. Hyperglycaemia in pregnancy can cause foetal abnormalities. Although the care of mothers with diabetes and their babies has improved dramatically over the last twenty years, perinatal mortality rates are still much higher in pregnancies where the mother has diabetes than where she has not (Audit Commission 2000).

Type 2 (or non-insulin dependent) diabetes

Type 2 diabetes is a metabolic disorder in which changes in the body's cells cause insulin resistance. It is associated with obesity and a sedentary lifestyle and usually appears in adults over 40. It is one of Britain's most common chronic diseases and is a leading cause of early death. At present diabetes affects at least 1.4 million people in the UK (3 per cent of the population) although it is thought that a further 1 million may be undiagnosed (Turner 1998). Like type 1 diabetes, it is increasing in incidence. The European Association for the Study of Diabetes predicts that the number of new cases of diabetes worldwide will double to 270 million people by 2010, of whom 4 million will be British (Dyer 2002).

The trend in obesity in British children and their lack of exercise has been blamed for the appearance of type 2 diabetes in adolescents. Although type 2 has previously been identified in children of Asian and African origin who are at higher risk, a number of white British teenagers, all of whom were overweight, have recently been diagnosed (Drake *et al.* 2002). It is expected that the incidence of type 2 diabetes will increase in parallel with the growing rate of childhood obesity which has doubled among British children in the last twenty years. In the United States the incidence of type 2 diabetes has been called an 'epidemic'. In 1999, for example, type 2 accounted for up to 45 per cent of new cases of childhood diabetes depending on locality (Kaufman 2002). This relatively new incidence of younger onset of type 2 diabetes is of great concern as young sufferers will be at a similar risk of medical complications to adults with type 2 diabetes.

MODY (maturity onset diabetes of the young)

MODY is a rare genetic form of diabetes arising from an inherited mutated gene. To date five genes have been identified that account for 80 per cent of the very few people in the UK who have this condition (Shepherd *et al.* 2001).

A cure for diabetes?

Although there is currently no cure for diabetes, there are a number of ongoing research programmes which aim to reduce the need for people with diabetes to be reliant on injected insulin. These include studies that involve converting cells from one type to another, islet transplantation and pancreatic transplant. Research projects also focus on more traditional treatments. These include the development of less invasive forms of insulin delivery such as insulin pumps and non-injection insulin delivery devices.

3. The diabetes services

Guidelines for the care of young people and the National Service Framework for Diabetes (DH 2001) favour a 'structured' and 'smooth' transfer to adult care for young people with diabetes. A national survey of paediatricians caring for children and young people with diabetes carried out in 1998 (Jefferson *et al.* 2003) found that just over half of respondents (52 per cent) had organised age stratified clinics and nearly all of these (95 per cent) were either an adolescent or a young adult clinic. The ages at which young people made the move to adult care varied between 14 and 20 years. In 14 per cent of cases young people were aged 14 to 16 years, in 31 per cent cases they were 16 and in 45 per cent between 16 and 20. Only 2 per cent of paediatricians reported that age at handover occurred in response to patient preference.

The diabetes services included in this study represent different arrangements for the care of young people and, particularly, for their transition to adult care. A typology of transfer arrangements was drawn up with the help of data from the survey mentioned above (Jefferson *et al.* 2003) and with advice from the director of Diabetes UK's National Paediatric Audit. The typology includes the different components of transition arrangements offered by different hospitals. However, although the categories broadly describe different arrangements, they are not mutually exclusive. Hospitals might have a staged approach to transition which could include an adolescent clinic based in the paediatric department, a clinic for older adolescents jointly run by paediatric and adult staff, and a dedicated clinic for young adults run by adult services. Other hospitals might only offer one or two of these components.

The arrangements at most hospitals are covered by the following typology:

- a young adolescent clinic based in the paediatric department;
- a joint clinic run by staff from both paediatric and adult services for young people before transfer to adult care;

- a young adult clinic run by the adult service;
- a diabetes service located in a dedicated adolescent unit;
- a letter at handover from the paediatric service to the adult service;
- no formal handover as adult diabetologists care for both children and adults;
- transition varies as a children's hospital transfers care to a number of adult services based in local hospitals.

Many hospitals offer some kind of specialised service at transition but there are other factors that differentiate services. The age at which young people make the transition varies, for example, as does the length of time they can attend the transition clinic. Some hospitals have a dedicated diabetes centre or department while in others clinics are run in outpatient departments. Multidisciplinary hospital teams also vary in size and make-up. Some, for example, offer dietetic advice to young people at every clinic appointment while others do not have adequate staff to make this possible. Diabetes specialist nurses who have been paediatrically trained are employed by some but not all trusts. Results from the survey of paediatricians mentioned above (Jefferson *et al.* 2003) showed that, although a majority of specialist nurses had undertaken training in paediatric diabetes, many did not specialise solely in this area. The availability of a psychology service where young people can be referred also varies as does access to podiatry.

Routine screening undertaken at every clinic appointment is also variable although the large majority measure HbA1c (glycated haemoglobin) at all clinic appointments. People with diabetes are encouraged to check their blood sugar levels regularly as an immediate guide to daily decision making about insulin dose and food intake as blood sugar levels fluctuate all the time. Measuring 'glycated haemoglobin' (called haemoglobin A1c or HbA1c) checks the amount of glucose attached to the haemoglobin inside the red blood cells. Red blood cells live for eight to 12 weeks so measuring HbA1c gives an average blood sugar level over this period. It is a useful way of telling whether diabetes is well controlled as a higher percentage result means that more glucose is attached to the haemoglobin. Over a longer period, consecutive HbA1c tests show a trend in overall diabetes control which can be used by the person with diabetes and their doctor to make decisions about treatment and to set goals for improvement. Other screening procedures include checking weight, height, blood pressure, thyroid function, lipids, renal function, full blood count, liver function, retinopathy and neuropathy screening and screening for coeliac disease. Some screening procedures are carried out at every appointment while others are done annually or every two years depending on the individual patient's age and the duration of diabetes.

In order to examine how clinics displaying differing transition arrangements operate, the six diabetes services included in the study were selected because they have different systems for transferring young people from paediatric to adult care. Four are located in district general hospitals, one in a children's hospital and the other in a teaching hospital. The hospitals serve diverse populations.

The research sites

The choice of sites for this study was made with the primary aim of including services with differing transition arrangements. Other factors were the wish to involve hospitals that served diverse communities, caseload sizes and areas of Britain. A shortlist was drawn up using data supplied by Diabetes UK (Jefferson *et al.* 2003), responses from health care professionals to short pieces in *Diabetes Update* and the *Journal of Diabetes Nursing*, as well as suggestions made by the project's advisory group members. It was also necessary to be pragmatic when choosing sites as it was important that health care staff were willing and had the capacity to participate. Staff at two hospitals declined to be involved because of existing local research projects, feeling that it would not be appropriate to ask young respondents to help with further research.

The six research sites selected are diverse across a number of variables and reflect the differing approaches to transition taken across a larger sample of hospitals. The hospital in area E, for example, is a city children's hospital with the largest caseload of young people with diabetes in Britain. Young people are referred on to a number of district hospitals and it is not logistically possible to offer formalised transition arrangements in collaboration with each of these. The hospital in area C, on the other hand, is a district hospital serving a largely rural population where children's and adult services are both located in the same building, making a joint clinic run by paediatric and adult staff relatively simple to arrange. With a sample of six, it is of course not possible to be representative of all types of hospital or of transition arrangements. However, the geographical spread, the different communities served, caseload sizes and the diverse arrangements at transition mean that the chosen sites give the study the opportunity to provide insights into the differing experiences of young people making use of these services.

Staff members at each of the hospitals included in the study were interviewed in order to investigate how the arrangements for transfer worked in both theory and practice as well as to throw light upon the team's philosophy in relation to the care of adolescents more generally. The history of local transition arrangements, the relationship between paediatric and adult services and any aspirations staff members had for developing services for adolescents and young adults were explored as were the constraints encountered. Doctors, nurses and dieticians from both paediatric and adult departments, one psychologist and one coordinator of diabetes services participated in interviews. In some hospitals it was not possible to interview all team members because of their busy schedules and, in some cases, the interviews were brief because of the demands of clinical work. In all 31 members of staff were interviewed.

Members of clinic staff were asked to comment on the development of the service in their hospital, current arrangements and plans for the future. Details about each clinic, therefore, provide a snapshot of the service at a particular time and are not a formal evaluation of clinic practice. The descriptions given below are taken from data provided by interviews with participating staff. Like all the information derived from interviews with both staff and young people, these are coloured by the perceptions and views of respondents.

Detailed information on service provision for young people was collected from hospital staff. This included the timing of and staffing arrangements for clinics, numbers of patients seen at clinics, tests routinely undertaken, protocols for non-attendance and policy and practice concerning transfer from paediatric to adult services. Changes in provision over the period of a year and new developments were included in order to map services over time. The interview schedule for staff was semi-structured, allowing researchers to ask about local circumstances, plans for developing transition services, and relationships with other services such as psychology, and with ward staff and staff at other local hospitals in cases where young people are transferred to another hospital. The interviews were tape recorded and transcribed. Data was analysed using the NVivo qualitative computer software package.

It must be noted that clinic arrangements alone do not constitute a diabetes service for young people. The service should also comprise home visits, school visits, education programmes, support between appointments and special projects. Diabetes care outside the clinic is explored in Chapter 5 and education in Chapters 11 and 12.

Research site A

This research site is in an outer London borough situated to the north-east of the City of London. Both paediatric and adult diabetes services are based in a district general hospital. There are also community clinics run in GPs' surgeries with support from diabetes specialist nurses.

The adolescent clinic

Hospital caseload size
154 patients aged 0–16

Ages of patients at transfer
Paediatric clinic → Adolescent clinic: age 13
Adolescent clinic → Adult clinic: age 17

Clinics
Frequency: Monthly
Time: 4 p.m.–6 p.m.
Number of patients per clinic: 6
Patients attend every 4 months
Location: Outpatients department

The diabetes team
Consultant paediatrician
Consultant physician (adult service)
Two diabetes specialist nurses (paediatric and adult services)
Paediatric dietician

Development of the adolescent service

When the paediatric diabetes specialist nurse came into post in 1996, part of her role was to develop a service for adolescents. At the time the children's clinic was over-subscribed and the paediatrician was moving patients as young as 13 to adult services in order to manage the caseload. The adult diabetologist, the newly appointed paediatric specialist nurse and one of the specialist nurses for adults developed the adolescent clinic. They believed that a dedicated clinic for young people was an important component of good diabetes care and, despite limited support from colleagues, decided to go ahead and set up a clinic for this age group.

Initially the adolescent clinic ran as an unacknowledged 'extra'. It was under-resourced with no administrative support so the two nurses involved had to 'pull' the notes themselves as well as act as receptionist and clinic nurse. There were also problems with patients not being entered onto the administrative system so that booking appointments and keeping records of test results was a problem. More recently there has been a change in how services are structured and the administrative work is now carried out routinely in the way other clinics are serviced although the paediatric nurse admitted that 'there are lots of glitches along the way'. Another improvement has been the presence of the paediatric consultant at clinics. When the clinic was first developed, it was assumed that there would be a paediatrician involved but this has only recently been achieved.

The ages of young people

Young people are referred to the adolescent clinic at 13 and then move up to the adult clinic at the time of their seventeenth birthday. Initially the plan was to see young people aged 13 to 16 but the clinic is popular and, in order to allow them more time before being referred to adult services, it was agreed that they could attend until the age of 17. This is not seen as ideal by staff who feel they would like to extend the service to patients older than 17 but is manageable with the limited resources available. At present it would not be possible to retain the small size of the clinic and allow those over 17 to continue attending. There is some flexibility in the age band seen. In some cases, patients younger than 13 are referred to the clinic because they are particularly mature for their age but sometimes there is a delay in referring them on:

> We've had a few young people that have been a bit delayed
> in being referred up and they look like sore pins in the
> paediatric department, you know, these great lumps.
> *(Paediatric diabetes specialist nurse)*

Frequency, timing and size of the adolescent clinic

The clinics run monthly and are scheduled from four till six o'clock in the evening in order to encourage young people who are studying or working to attend. There is provision for an extra clinic every quarter and occasionally extra clinics are fitted in if the caseload is particularly large at one time. Young people attend every four months. The clinic is small with only six (or sometimes seven) patients booked in each month.

The staff team

As noted above, the adolescent clinic has limited resources. It is staffed by a consultant diabetologist from the adult service and two diabetes specialist nurses, one paediatric and one adult. Recently a consultant paediatrician has joined the team which will make it more like a genuine transition clinic allowing young people to have the continuity of consulting with a physician and a nurse whom they already know while giving them the opportunity to meet and get to know staff from the adult diabetes service. Another new addition is a paediatric dietician who has recently been employed by the hospital trust.

The team who staff the adolescent clinic is therefore mixed, coming from both adult and paediatric diabetes services. The paediatric nurse was positive about the way the team works together although she admitted that sometimes there can be problems over areas of responsibility between paediatric and adult services at the point at which young people make the transition. This may be an issue if young people who have been attending the teenage clinic under the care of the adult diabetologist are admitted to hospital and placed in a paediatric ward where they will see the consultant paediatrician.

> I think we work really well, and a part of it is that the adult
> diabetes team has allowed me to join their team, you know,
> they always had a good team, so they see me as part of that
> team, so I go on away days with them and stuff so I do feel
> that we are. I think it comes across that we're a team and
> that we get on and that we all work in similar ways.
> *(Paediatric diabetes specialist nurse)*

The team is coordinated by one of the nurses who organises dates and clinic arrangements and reminds members of staff and young people to attend. The whole diabetes team meets monthly and this is an opportunity for discussion about aspects of the service. Informal discussion between clinics is also an important element in ensuring that the service runs smoothly, that young people are followed up and that any issues about individuals' care are aired.

As is the case with all but one of the diabetes services included in the study, there is not a psychologist in the team but nurses do refer young people with psychological problems to Child and Adolescent Mental Health Services. Staff would prefer some input from a psychologist as routine but this service is not currently available.

What I feel is there should be someone there right from the beginning to meet the family as part of the team, so that it's not seen as abnormal, but at the moment it's still a bit 'hit crisis, refer'… Every other one of my patients seems to have some emotional crisis going on and you try your best to talk through it with them, but we don't have the entire skills to deal with it.
(Paediatric diabetes specialist nurse)

Clinic structure

The most significant difference between the paediatric and adolescent clinics is their size. Six patients are booked for each adolescent clinic which is a much smaller number than in either paediatric or adult clinics although at some seven are booked because there is a larger than usual cohort of patients in the age group. This small number gives the young people attending the opportunity to have more time to discuss issues with members of staff as well as reducing waiting times. Young people have an individual one-to-one consultation and, because of smaller numbers, there is more choice about whether parents sit in at the meeting with the doctor, nurse or dietician. When the young person comes into the clinic, they first see the nurse from the adult service who will carry out routine screening. They will then have the opportunity to consult with the nurse about their diabetes control and anything else they may want to talk about. The nurse will ask them to check their blood glucose level to ensure that they are using their equipment correctly.

So the consultation with the nurse serves two purposes really. Things that need to be addressed in between times and things that need to be immediately addressed in their medical consultation and that bit obviously includes the surveillance.
(Diabetes specialist nurse – adult service)

Although there is a set structure for a clinic attendance, nurses take a flexible approach.

We've got a clinic sheet that we sort of go through and often it's not formal, you know, I follow it but you often follow a different path and let the doctor do all the formal bits because you might have started talking about school and what's happened at school.
(Paediatric diabetes specialist nurse)

Whether or not nurses have identified any problems or issues that need attention, each young person consults with the doctor and also gets the opportunity to talk to the dietician.

The atmosphere in the clinic is intended to be fairly informal although care is shown by nurses to ensure privacy for young people, particularly when they are being weighed. Both nurses said it was difficult to initiate communication between young people while they were waiting and no formal education or group sessions have been organised. Although parents chat, young patients are uncomfortable about talking to each other.

> We try and make it really interactive and sit amongst them and have a chat with them and, you know, try and get the parents talking – you can't get the kids talking to each other however hard you try.
> *(Paediatric diabetes specialist nurse)*

One of the nurses has produced a display board which she updates regularly with relevant information on new developments in diabetes care. This can act as a focal point for patients.

> It sometimes happens that somebody will ask about something on the board which is obviously relevant for everybody so people will also get involved so it happens spontaneously but we haven't done anything formal. We'd like to but the reality of teenage life is that anything that you try and organise isn't necessarily what they like.
> *(Diabetes specialist nurse – adult service)*

Screening

Young people are weighed and their height measured and their blood pressure checked routinely at each clinic they attend. Blood glucose levels over a three-month period are also measured (the HbA1c test) at each clinic appointment. Screening for thyroid and renal function, lipids and a full blood count is also carried out. Liver function is also checked at intervals.

> We do more tests there. With the paediatric clinic we don't do the blood test, not in clinic, or the wee test, but we do tend to with the adolescents. Part of getting them to test their blood is more a learning thing to see what technique they're using, whether they're using their meters properly,

because we get them to bring their own so that's why we do it, not that we believe a one-off random test gives you any information but it is a learning thing, and so another point of intervention. And the wee test is really to check for protein and stuff, and to check if they've got ketones.
(Paediatric diabetes specialist nurse)

Location

The hospital does not have a dedicated diabetes centre and clinics are held in the outpatients department. Staff do not feel this is an ideal setting and are unable to make it inviting by, for example, playing music, because there are other clinics running nearby at the same time. Both nurses who were interviewed put a more welcoming environment high on the list of improvements they would like to make.

It's an awful outpatients department anyway, I mean for anybody, but yeah, I mean it's still very much a hospital clinic, you know. There's still a few other clinics going on so we couldn't put music on or, you know, have snooker or anything like that because it's just not that sort of environment. There's nowhere where they can make tea or coffee. It's dull and dreary.
(Paediatric diabetes specialist nurse)

It's not ideal at all although, because there are only a few people, that helps. It's a traditional clinic, it's definitely a hospital, it's definitely got rooms behind closed doors although recently it looks much better because it is the children's floor so obviously a number of them have got younger brothers and sisters so it's actually quite good for them. There's plenty for them to do while they're waiting so it's quite good from a family point of view but, no, it's not ideal. It doesn't lend itself to discussions because there is that sense of hospital formality and I don't think you can get away from that. The place is being used by lots of other people all the time and it's not ours and I think ownership's important, we don't feel it's ours and see it very much as 'the hospital', so not mad about it but it's not bad because the numbers are small.
(Diabetes specialist nurse – adult service)

Future plans

The adolescent clinic was set up with very limited resources in terms of staffing and administrative support but is now well established due to the enthusiasm and commitment of members of staff from both paediatric and adult services keen to offer appropriate care for teenagers. Despite what one nurse called the 'DIY' nature of its beginnings, it has developed since its initiation in 1996. Information systems have improved, the team has expanded to include a consultant paediatrician and a dietician, and young people are able to attend until their seventeenth birthday. In order to make further improvements, staff would like to meet with users of the service to discuss with them how changes might be made for the better. The availability of a psychologist as part of the multidisciplinary team was also identified as something that might be considered for the future.

Both nurses would like to improve the clinic environment and one was keen to be able to provide a drop-in system for young people. Creating a dedicated diabetes centre or dedicated department with attractive surroundings would be, however, an expensive development.

> I'd definitely like a better environment. Where there can be a drop-in arrangement as well because some of the people who don't come can't, it's just not at the right time. Why should the right time for us make it the right time for them? And perhaps at the end of the day after a long day at school the last thing they want is more school effectively, so to have an arrangement where people could come when they needed to – that's true for the whole diabetes service – it would be brilliant.
> *(Diabetes specialist nurse – adult service)*

> I'd like a nicer environment to make it a bit more sort of relaxed really, yeah, comfy chairs. You know, it's very much school chairs. If we had a diabetes centre I have images of like a club atmosphere with music, obviously not wild music, but, you know, snooker or having the telly on. I think the environment is important to teenagers. If they think they're coming to a fun place they actually might come.
> *(Paediatric diabetes specialist nurse)*

Nurses were also keen to ensure the service is focused on the age group targeted. There is no particular specialist in adolescence in the team and they would like this to be addressed. New developments tend to be initiated by the paediatric diabetes specialist nurse and she feels the burden of responsibility for convening clinics and all the other practical tasks involved in running the service. Sometimes that means that there is limited time to discuss and try out new developments in the service although she described the team as one that communicates well.

> I would like to see more cohesive teams I suppose, but hopefully we're working towards that. We could try and make it more teenaged, perhaps people that have a bit more training in working with adolescents. For example, recently there's been talk of having one of the health care assistants who's taken a particular interest in adolescents to come and work in the clinic. It's a different culture. It's easy to see them as the bad, bad bunch and you often talk about the bad things with teenagers but there are some that just get on and do it and evolve through their teens without any problems, so you need to be very level-headed, understanding, understand social issues, you know, have some information about drugs, about sexual health, so many things.
> *(Paediatric diabetes specialist nurse)*

Another interest is in setting up a young adult clinic which adolescents could move on to when they are 17 but, again, there are resource constraints.

> We'd love to do that, it just isn't possible with the current service resources. There isn't the space to plan it apart from anything else but obviously that's an ideal situation because people are more sociable at that age and it's much more likely that they'll find the group bit of it more valuable. So we would love to do that. That's the difference in the adult clinic because they don't all come at the same time, so you sort of lose that sense of belonging to a group, so, yeah, we'd really like to age band throughout, but it's more complicated than it sounds.
> *(Diabetes specialist nurse – adult service)*

Research site B

The service is based in a city in the north of England where there is a diverse population which includes a large South Asian community. Children's diabetes services are based in one hospital, which has a paediatric department, and young people move to the diabetes department in another hospital for transition and adult care. The diabetes service has benefited from extra funding under the Health Action Zone initiative and this has allowed an extra paediatric diabetes nurse to be employed and been used to fund holidays for children with diabetes.

The transition clinic

Hospital caseload size
145 patients aged 0–16

Ages of patients at transfer
Paediatric clinic ➔ Adolescent clinic: age 14
Adolescent clinic ➔ Transition clinic: age 16 (after taking GCSEs)
Transition clinic ➔ Adult clinic: age 17

Clinics
Frequency: Three monthly
Time: 5 p.m.–6.30 p.m.
Number of patients per clinic: Varies from 10 to more than 15 depending on size of cohort
Patients attend every 3 months
Location: Hospital diabetes department

The diabetes team
Consultant paediatrician
Consultant physician (adult service)
Two diabetes specialist nurses (paediatric and adult services)
Dietician (adult service)

Development of the adolescent service

The 'transition clinic' as it is known was initiated by staff from the paediatric department at one of the city's hospitals. There had been some resistance to the idea from the adult side but personnel changes meant that paediatric staff saw their opportunity and began running the clinic as an experimental service in 1998. The clinic allows young people to transfer from the paediatric department in one hospital to the diabetes department in another where adult services are based while keeping contact with staff they already know. This gives them the chance to familiarise themselves with the new environment and adult staff before they transfer to adult services. The clinic is run by staff from both paediatric and adult teams.

The ages of young people

Before moving up to the transition clinic, teenagers aged 14 to 16 attend an 'adolescent clinic' based in the paediatric department. They move to the transition clinic in the September after they have completed their GCSE exams. All those who have finished studying for GCSEs move together aged 16 years, although some will be just 16 while others will be approaching their seventeenth birthday. They remain in that clinic for a year and are transferred to the adult service the following September. Moving young people up together means that they will remain with the same cohort as they progress to the adult clinic.

> We run our clinics very much based on the school year so we start our clinics in September as it were and so young folk tend to move around with their school peer group, in their school year.
> *(Consultant paediatrician)*

The advantage of age banding means that clinic staff are able to focus on the particular issues raised by young people who have finished their statutory schooling and are either studying for further qualifications or have started work. Some will have moved from school to tertiary education. One nurse expressed her concern that young people can only attend the transition clinic for one year and thought it should perhaps run for two until young people who are studying have finished their A-levels and reached the age of 18 but at present limited resources mean that it is not possible to extend the service.

Frequency, timing and size of the adolescent clinic

Clinics are run every three months in the early evening, from 5 p.m. to 6.30 p.m., to ensure attendance does not interfere with study or work. The number of young people booked for each clinic depends on the size of the cohort who have diabetes in that particular age group. The numbers fluctuate from between ten to more than 15.

> Last year we only had about nine in the transition clinic. This year we've got something like 16 or 17. It's a big clinic this time because the ones that are in the transition clinic were born in 1984 and for some reason that was a bumper year for us! They weren't all diagnosed at the same time at the same age but it is a very big group. So we've actually had to transfer about 16. We're going to get more like that. It's going to be pretty similar each year. The numbers might vary between 12 and 18, but it's going to be over ten.
> *(Paediatric diabetes specialist nurse)*

The staff team

The transition clinic is run jointly by paediatric and adult services in the diabetes department where adults are cared for. There are two consultants, one a paediatrician who already knows the young people attending, and one a diabetologist who has the opportunity to get to know them before they are transferred to the adult service. Also in attendance are diabetes specialist nurses from both paediatric and adult services and a dietician. A podiatrist is available for referral.

Clinic structure

At clinic appointments young people see either the paediatrician or the adult physician. Originally the idea was that at their first appointment at the transition clinic patients would see both doctors together and in the following ones they would alternate and that the paediatrician might not need to attend the final clinic. This arrangement was not convenient, however, so young people see either one or the other consultant. The doctors try to ensure that they see different patients at each appointment.

Like the adolescent clinic described above in area A, the transition clinic has limited nurse support and the paediatric nurse present has restricted time to talk to each young person because she spends time on administration, paperwork and routine screening.

> Because of the restriction of staff, because it's in the evening and it's not staffed very well. If the other paediatric nurse or I are there, we tend to end up doing the bloods for the HbA1c's so we end up with this very technical role and not an awful lot of time to talk to the children because they're coming through on a conveyer belt so you're trying to get them through so that's done before they have their appointment. There isn't a clinic nurse on duty at that time and it's obviously not been funded for that so we end up doing it – complete waste of resources. It sounds ridiculous either a G or an H grade doing heights, weights and bloods but, yeah, that's just the way it is.
> *(Paediatric diabetes specialist nurse)*

The dietician cannot see all patients at every appointment so tries to ensure that she has a consultation with someone that she did not see at the last appointment.

Screening

An HbA1c blood test is taken at each clinic visit and results are immediately available. Young people are also weighed and, if they are still growing, measured. Eye screening is undertaken annually. Each patient has an annual review when they are screened for lipids, thyroid function, kidney function, liver function and coeliac disease.

One of the consultants described the usefulness of a routine HbA1c test in encouraging patients to make an extra effort with their glycaemic control because someone apart from themselves is taking an interest in their well-being. Like overweight patients with type 2 diabetes who are regularly weighed, he suggested that because the test is routinely administered with instant results young people are encouraged to 'pass' it.

> I think that role in terms of HbA1c applies as well. If they think somebody else is going to pay a bit of attention to it,

> cares what's happening to them, then it's worth making a bit
> of an effort. Externally imposed pressures are often more
> powerful than internally imposed ones. You can read a
> textbook just for your own education and it doesn't matter
> whether you take it in or not but if you've got to sit an exam
> at the end of it you're going to pay much more attention to it.
> *(Consultant diabetologist)*

Some young people might have a different view. Being expected to pass a test
may cause anxiety or even discourage young people who feel they cannot 'pass'
from attending the clinic.

Location

The transition clinic takes place in the diabetes department of the hospital
where adult diabetes services are located. The location is new to young people
who previously attended clinics in the children's outpatients department of a
different hospital in the city. It is also unfamiliar territory to the paediatric
consultant and nurses who help staff the clinic. The paediatrician was
concerned that young people would be put off by coming across much older
diabetes patients in the waiting room but this has not happened as the clinic
runs in the evening when there are no other clinics. Although it is run in a
dedicated diabetes unit, the paediatrician felt that this was probably not an
important consideration for young patients.

> I think the children's outpatients is a very friendly place.
> I think most of our long-term patients feel that and don't
> mind coming or like coming or whatever. I agree it's good
> to have a dedicated diabetes unit. I'm not sure what impact
> that has on our transition teenagers. I think they probably
> see it as somewhere a bit strange really rather than being
> especially friendly.
> *(Consultant paediatrician)*

Future plans

Like members of staff at clinic A, doctors and nurses at clinic B are keen to
develop the service they offer to young people in a way that is acceptable to
them. They are looking at options and are considering employing a diabetes

specialist nurse with responsibility for young people up to the age of 25 after they have made the transition to adult services. A nurse in this role would be able to offer a service to university students in the city. The nurse would ensure that contact is maintained with services and that young people would continue to be cared for even if they were unwilling to regularly attend clinic appointments. There is a particular concern that young people are not keen to be treated alongside much older people with diabetes who may have visible complications that young people do not want to be in contact with. In order to proceed, a case must be made to support the new initiative and funding agreed by the primary care trusts.

> Nationally it's recognised that there's a high drop-out rate
> from adult services by young people and our concerns really
> are to develop something for young people which will be
> acceptable to them so that they'll at least keep in contact
> and have a yearly health check and so on. We're not exactly
> clear how that will be offered or where it will be offered but
> our plan anyway is to try to have a diabetes specialist nurse
> particularly taking on the young people post- transition.
> *(Consultant paediatrician)*

Another concern is to offer care in surroundings where young people feel comfortable. There are 'satellite clinics' in the area where specially trained GPs provide diabetes services to adults and these might be an alternative to hospital care for some young adults who are unwilling or unable to attend hospital appointments. The relatively small numbers of young people, however, mean that it might not be a feasible option to offer transition clinics specifically for young people in local areas but it is something that is being considered.

> I just wonder if we should be doing the transition clinics in a
> different way and setting them up so maybe we can split the
> group into four so we do just one transition clinic or two
> transition clinics with a quarter of them, do it that way, but
> in a locality, like a medical centre or something, in a PCT.
> And involve a GP from a satellite clinic or do something. But
> something different. Whatever we are doing, I'm not happy
> with the format at the moment.
> *(Paediatric diabetes specialist nurse)*

Research site C

The diabetes service is based in a district general hospital in a county town serving a rural area in the south-west. There are a number of boarding schools in the area which boost the numbers of young people being cared for by hospital staff.

The young adult clinic

Hospital caseload size
40 patients aged 0–16

Ages of patients at transfer
Paediatric clinic ➔ Young adult clinic: age 16 or 17
Young adult clinic ➔ Adult clinic: age early 20s

Clinics
Frequency: Three monthly
Time: 2.45 p.m.–4.30 p.m.
Number of patients per clinic: 8 to 12
Patients attend every 3 to 6 months
Location: Outpatients department

The diabetes team
Paediatrician
Consultant physician (adult service)
One diabetes specialist nurse (paediatric and adult services)
Dietician (paediatric and adult services)

Development of the adolescent service

In this service, young people move from paediatric care to a clinic run jointly by the adult consultant and the paediatrician. There are no diabetes specialist nurses working only with children so continuity is also provided by the nurse who works with both children and adults.

The paediatrician described how she was prompted to consider a formalised transition service when she met one of her patients in the supermarket.

> I met one of my old patients in Tesco's who we diagnosed at
> the age of 18 months. He was then about 19, I suppose, and
> he'd been transferred under the old system which was when
> you got to 16 you had a letter and you went to see the adults
> and that was that, and they'd seen him once and he was
> beautifully controlled which he was, and had discharged him
> back to the GP's care and he was quite unhappy about that.
> And that really was it.
> *(Paediatrician)*

The transition clinic was set up in 1996 with support from both paediatric and
adult staff to provide a service for young people who may already have been
living with diabetes for a number of years but who did not fit the profile of
older adults attending the hospital clinic because they were not developing
diabetic complications. Young people diagnosed in their late teenage years and
who have never attended paediatric clinics are also referred to the young adult
clinic. Previously young people leaving paediatric care would have been referred
to the adult clinic by a letter from the paediatrician and one of the adult nurses
may have been invited to their last paediatric appointment in order to
introduce herself although this arrangement was not systematically adhered to.
If young people had no signs of complications they would have been referred to
their GP who would be unlikely to have specialist knowledge of type 1 diabetes
or of the particular issues facing young people living with the condition.

The ages of young people

Young people move from the paediatric to the young adult clinic at around 16 or
17 but the timing of the move can be flexible depending on the individual's
circumstances and needs. If a young person is coping with another medical
condition, he or she may also stay in the paediatric clinic until they are older
than 17.

> If they're going out to work at 16 we often transfer them.
> If they're staying on at college or school we may keep
> them until they're 17. It varies enormously.
> *(Diabetes specialist nurse)*

The hospital is a small trust so there are not enough patients to run dedicated
clinics for narrow age bands. For this reason, young people may continue to

attend the young adult clinic until they are in their early twenties, depending on their circumstances. The paediatrician has wide experience of working with adolescents and young adults and the clinic is oriented to their needs. It is understood by staff that adult care may not be appropriate for those who may be studying in another town or planning to travel abroad for a period and the clinic aims to provide a service for all those who may be leading lives that are not yet settled.

> I think the ethos in the adult world is very much adult orientated, you're now an adult, get on with it as if you were, and many of them are not at that stage, they're just not mature in many ways, and I think sometimes for the children with diabetes, all the ones who've come through childhood with diabetes, all those problems are compounded because the sort of breaking away process is quite difficult for them and just suddenly to be landed in an adult type environment...
> *(Diabetes specialist nurse)*

It is recognised, however, that some young people may prefer to break away from medical staff who have known them since they were much younger and seek diabetes care elsewhere, which they could do by going to a clinic in the town where they are studying or consulting their GP.

Frequency, timing and size of the adolescent clinic

Young adult clinics run every three or four months and are scheduled to coincide with university vacations so that students studying away from home can attend. They run in the afternoon between 2.45 p.m. and 4.30 p.m. There are fewer patients booked than in the adult clinics so waiting times are relatively short and there is time to discuss any concerns with staff.

> The whole clinic is geared to them and there'll be about seven or eight seen in a session which is a fraction of what is seen in the hurly-burly of the adult clinic.
> *(Consultant physician)*

However, numbers have been increasing because of caseload size and, recently, up to 12 young people are booked for each clinic. Each patient is allocated 15 minutes for their appointment but sometimes they need more which means waiting times may increase. Staff members suggested that there could be more clinics and for a longer period so that there would be more time to spend with young patients.

The staff team

The clinic is staffed by doctors from both children's and adult services, a diabetes specialist nurse and a dietician. Both the nurse and the dietician work with children and adults. There is a clinic nurse who greets patients, carries out administration tasks and weighs patients. There is no podiatrist routinely available although one of the doctors regularly checks patients' feet. One member of staff was concerned at the lack of psychological support.

> I think an area we're poor in is psychological care in terms of referrals to other professionals. It doesn't happen really. It does in the children's clinic if they've gone into the children's system, they may get more follow on care in young adult life but we don't seem to have much of a pathway for referral on to the psychologist.
> *(Diabetes specialist nurse)*

Clinic structure

When young people come to a clinic appointment, they are first weighed and then come into the consultation room where they meet with both doctors, the adult physician and the paediatrician, and the diabetes specialist nurse and dietician. If they have previously been to appointments in the paediatric department they will already know the paediatrician, nurse and dietician. The clinic is led by the adult physician who is the senior consultant but other staff members have the opportunity to join in with the consultation which is intended to be quite informal.

> We've got the adult physician in the big chair because this is grown ups and we no longer have Thomas the Tank Engine on the walls and all the rest of it, but it seems to work. We do interrupt and keep the ball rolling and keep it more of a sort of conversation, you know, there's certainly not a rigid turn and turn about and one would hope that a lot of the talking is actually going to come from the patient.
> *(Paediatrician)*

There are advantages and disadvantages to this arrangement. On one hand, seeing the staff team together makes the time spent in the clinic shorter and means that greetings and explanations do not need to be repeated. Staff in all hospitals reported that on the whole young people want to spend as short a time as possible in the clinic. The fact that some staff members know the patient well also allows the team to have a brief update about a particular person before they come into the room. From staff members' point of view, it is useful to know how other professionals approach issues and helps to make a cohesive team. On the other hand, it could be intimidating for someone to come into a room and be faced with four professionals even though they are likely to know at least two of them quite well. However, this arrangement is also used in the paediatric clinic and so is something young people are used to. Advice is not restricted to time spent at clinic appointments. Both the dietician and the diabetes specialist nurse are willing to make extra appointments between clinics to discuss particular concerns and they work together closely to support patients.

Screening

At each clinic appointment patients are weighed and their blood pressure monitored. There is no on-site facility for testing blood for HbA1c so patients are asked to send in a blood sample by post two weeks before their appointment. If they do so results will be available at the appointment. If they fail to do this, a blood sample will be taken at the appointment. Once a year blood and urine samples are screened for thyroid function, lipids and renal function. Blood pressure is checked annually or more often. Screening for coeliac disease is carried out every two to three years. Eyes are screened annually by local optometrists.

Location

The clinic is held in the outpatients department which staff feel is not an ideal setting but there is no dedicated diabetes unit at the hospital. At one time, the diabetes specialist nurse attempted to make the clinic atmosphere more sociable by providing drinks and snacks and chatted informally to those young people waiting. It was not a success as young people made it clear that they preferred not to interact with their peers and wanted to get the appointment over as quickly as possible.

Future plans

The adult clinic at the hospital is generally attended by older people who have medical problems associated with diabetes. These patients do not attend routine hospital follow-up appointments because their GPs take that role. Staff would like to extend the young adult clinic by introducing a clinic for those up to age 30 or 35 where the emphasis would continue to be on monitoring glycaemic control and giving advice on diet and lifestyle rather than on treating complications.

Research site D

The diabetes service has its own centre in the grounds of a district general hospital in an East Anglian town.

The teenage clinic

Hospital caseload size
185 patients aged 0–16

Ages of patients at transfer
Paediatric clinic ➜ Teenage clinic: age 12–14
Teenage clinic ➜ Adult clinic: age approximately 18

Clinics
Frequency: Three monthly
Time: 4 p.m.–6.30 p.m.
Number of patients per clinic: 12
Location: Diabetes centre

The diabetes team
Consultant paediatrician
Two consultant physicians (adult service)
Two diabetes specialist nurses (paediatric and adult services)
Diabetes specialist dietician

Development of the adolescent service

The arrangements in this service are unusual because adult physicians care for children with diabetes as well as teenagers and adults. This system developed because of a number of factors. In the early 1980s, when paediatric diabetes care emphasised children's social development and focused less on glycaemic control than is now the case, young people were transferred to adult services in their teenage years where the philosophy of care was very different and where clinics were much larger.

> What we found was that these kids came across with the
> message that now [doctors will] really tighten up on your
> diabetes and they came across in mid-puberty with this sort
> of threat and arrived in what was actually a very
> unsatisfactory diabetic clinic, as we still had the old
> fashioned sort of monster clinic, and you spent the next year
> cooling them down and trying to persuade them that
> actually you were quite friendly and getting them on track.
> *(Consultant diabetologist)*

The paediatrician who was looking after children with diabetes asked the adult diabetologist to assist him with his clinical work. This arrangement was agreed and they had joint consultations with children and their families. Eventually, because of time considerations and growing numbers of patients, they began to see patients separately. The hospital was one of the first to employ a diabetes specialist nurse early in the 1980s and she took responsibility for the nursing care of children. In the mid-1980s a dedicated diabetes centre was opened in the hospital grounds and the specialist nurse was based there and, in order to maintain continuity of care, it was agreed that children's diabetes clinics would be held in the new centre with the paediatrician in attendance. Young people attend a teenage clinic and continue to see the adult physicians whom they may have known for many years.

The ages of young people

Young people move to the teenage clinic when they are between 12 and 14 and stay until they are about 18. There is flexibility about when young people move but they are introduced to the idea of transferring to the teenage clinic when they are about 11 and make the move when they or members of staff feel they are ready to do so. Sometimes young people attend an adult clinic because they are unable to make it to the teenage clinic and may decide to continue to attend the adult clinic because the time is convenient. There is an adult clinic aimed at working people which is run at a time when it is possible for them to attend.

> It just happens they can't come up on that occasion [to the teenage clinic] and then they realise actually it's quite OK to come to the adult clinic. Not a problem. And again that adult clinic tends to be people who are working so it tends not to be very old people with difficulties.
> *(Consultant diabetologist)*

Frequency, timing and size of the adolescent clinic

Teenage clinics are held every three months in the afternoon and run until 6.30 or 7 p.m. to allow people who are working or studying to attend. Approximately 12 people are booked for each clinic.

The staff team

As noted above, adult doctors based in the diabetes centre care for children and young people. The teenage clinic is staffed by two consultant diabetologists, three diabetes specialist nurses and a dietician who specialises in diabetes. At most clinics there are also one or two senior house officers or registrars who also see patients. A paediatrically trained diabetes specialist nurse has recently been appointed and plans to work with young people as well as children although the caseload is large.

The diabetes centre also employs a play therapist who works mainly with younger children but, in some cases, with teenagers who are experiencing problems. Staff felt that the unavailability of an accessible and effective psychological service was a deficiency.

Clinic structure

When young people arrive at the clinic, they are first weighed and measured and blood samples are taken by one of the health care assistants. This is done in the centre's laboratory where there is some privacy. The newly appointed paediatric diabetes specialist nurse coordinates the clinic and makes sure patients are booked to see the doctor of their choice. Young people can choose whether they want to see the doctor alone or with their parent; sometimes a young person will consult with the doctor alone first and then their parent will join them. The dietician is available for anyone who wants advice from her and patients may use the consultation to ask a quick question or spend more time discussing dietary issues in detail.

Screening

Young people are weighed and their height and HbA1c measured. Eye screening, foot checks and other screening procedures are carried out annually.

Location

As noted above, the teenage clinic is held in the diabetes centre which is located in the hospital grounds but housed in a separate one storey building. The surroundings are more comfortable than an outpatients clinic and the space has the advantage of being dedicated to diabetes care. As one of the doctors put it: 'This belongs to diabetes. This is their unit.'

Future plans

A number of those interviewed talked about how they would like to improve the service for young people although, like staff in other hospitals, it is difficult to make time to discuss and develop innovations. There is concern about following up young people who fail to attend appointments because at the time of the interviews there was limited time available for home visits.

> I think we all know that we are not giving them the best
> deal. I think we're all lovely people and I think when they
> come and say 'help' they get it, but a lot of them don't come
> and say 'help' and it may be those that we need to address.
> *(Diabetes specialist nurse)*

There is a hope that the appointment of the new paediatric diabetes specialist nurse will be a catalyst for change in the service. Another area of interest is support and counselling for parents of children and teenagers with diabetes.

A voluntary organisation that provides counselling for couples will be based in the centre on an experimental basis to work with particular families who are experiencing problems. At the time of the interviews, this service had not yet begun. If the service is popular with families, it is hoped that some of the counsellors will offer training to medical staff to allow them to learn some of the skills involved in working with families.

Research site E

The diabetes service for children is located in a children's hospital in this Scottish city. It has the largest caseload of children with diabetes in Britain.

The adolescent clinic

Hospital caseload size
400 patients aged 0–15

Ages of patients at transfer
Paediatric clinic ➔ Adolescent clinic: age 12
Adolescent clinic ➔ Adult clinic: age 15

Clinics
Frequency: Weekly
Time: 4 p.m.–6 p.m.
Number of patients per clinic: 10
Patients attend every 4 months
Location: Outpatients department

The diabetes team
Consultant paediatrician
Staff grade physician
Three paediatric diabetes specialist nurses
Two paediatric dieticians

Development of the adolescent service

Children with diabetes are referred from all over the city and from surrounding areas including some rural areas many miles from the hospital. Children of all ages with diabetes are cared for and the service runs an adolescent clinic for those of 12 and over. When they reach the age of 15, young people are referred to adult services. Before 1993 the upper age limit was only 14 but it was agreed that this was too young an age to leave paediatric care. However, the raising of the age limit and the increase in incidence of type 1 diabetes has meant that the overall caseload size has continued to rise. When young people reach 15, they are referred to another hospital service in the locality where they live. Because young people are referred on to a large number of local hospitals, it is not possible to provide a jointly run transition service although, in the past, consultants from both the children's hospital and one of the adult services based in a local hospital worked together to provide a transition clinic.

> That did used to happen but for logistical reasons it fell
> through. It was only with one of the centres as well.
> *(Consultant paediatrician)*

The clinic was abandoned because of the difficulties of timetabling, staff availability and ensuring the service was convenient for patients and well attended enough to justify its existence.

The ages of young people

The adolescent clinic is aimed at 12 to 15 year olds but the age band is not strict and young people are moved from the children's to the adolescent clinic when it seems most appropriate for them.

> We say age 12, but there are some far more mature under 12
> year olds, and, being sexist, I have to say it's the girls that are
> more mature than the boys at that age, but if we felt that
> someone was particularly mature we would move them to
> the adolescent clinic before that, and if there was somebody
> that we felt was really young, it might be nearer when they're
> 13 before they would move over. But by the time they're 13
> they would definitely be at the adolescent clinic.
> *(Diabetes services coordinator)*

As noted above, the children's service is not available for young people over 15 years. Although staff would like to be able to extend the service above that age, it is not currently possible because of the large caseload.

> Age is the main criteria, because we'd love to keep them on for longer, but we're simply bursting at the seams.
> *(Diabetes services coordinator)*

> Eighteen would be a much better age probably to keep people to because you're only just beginning to see the problems of acceptance and things, you know, by the mid-teens and very often we feel like we're passing the buck onto our adult colleagues.
> *(Diabetes specialist nurse)*

In exceptional cases, there is flexibility in this arrangement.

> There is a little [flexibility] and it's entirely at my discretion. Nobody's forcing me to throw them out but the reality is that for every one that we keep on, that's an extra one on the books and we don't have the resources for what we've got. The kind of compelling reason would be a teenager who has been having a lot of problems and is showing willingness to change and needs help through that period. We may keep them a bit longer. We've had two or three children with other illnesses who are being managed by my other colleagues and we try and coordinate their transfers.
> *(Consultant paediatrician)*

Frequency, timing and size of the adolescent clinic

The weekly adolescent clinic runs on a weekday morning and approximately ten young people are booked in. They attend a clinic appointment every four months.

The staff team

The team is made up of a consultant paediatrician, a staff grade physician, one full-time and one part-time dietician and three diabetes specialist nurses. Other doctors also help with the clinic. Young people may not always see the same members of staff but, because the team is small, it is likely that they will get to know everybody. Each patient has a designated specialist nurse and they usually see that nurse at appointments. One nurse felt that it can be helpful for patients to see different members of staff.

> Personally I don't think it's desirable for them to see the
> same person all the time because sometimes new or
> different ideas from different people coming in at a
> different angle can shed new light onto somebody's
> particular problems.
> *(Paediatric diabetes specialist nurse)*

The diabetes service coordinator took a holistic view of who she considered part
of the diabetes team. A psychologist and social worker are not part of the core
team and do not routinely attend clinics but they are available for referrals.

> There's diabetes nurse specialists, and there's the consultant,
> the staff grade doctor, there's myself who's the diabetes
> coordinator and dietician, and the wider team includes the
> psychologist, and we did have a social worker who regularly
> attended but because they're so stretched it's really on a
> crisis only basis. I very much see the ward staff as members
> of the team too, and the GPs and … I mean schools, you
> know, wherever the child is, to me, they've got to be involved
> in the child's diabetes.
> *(Diabetes services coordinator)*

All members of staff who were interviewed were very positive about the team
itself, describing it as truly multidisciplinary with excellent communication
between members and a shared ethos. Although team members have their own
responsibilities and there is a hierarchy, staff felt that they knew each other well
and understood each other's roles.

> In regard to looking after the patients I think we do work very
> well together and it is quite cooperative. Although we have
> our own roles, everyone knows a bit about what everyone else
> is doing and I think we do communicate quite well.
> *(Paediatric diabetes specialist nurse)*

Another team member described how cohesive the team is both in terms of its
communication and the consistency of its approach.

> We never stop talking to each other! We do have a weekly
> meeting, and we will have informal meetings in between
> times and we share the same office and we're all
> geographically close so we do talk to each other a lot.

> We leave phone messages for each other, we leave notes for
> each other, and we e-mail each other! I think our strongest
> asset is that we work as a multidisciplinary team and we all
> work together and I think continuity and consistency is
> important, not only for us but even more so for the families.
> *(Diabetes services coordinator)*

Clinic structure

When young people attend the adolescent clinic from the age of 12 or 13, they
first have a consultation on their own and then their parents are asked to join
them. The team approach extends to the consultation itself where patients see
the doctor, dietician and nurse together. The reason young people are invited
to the consultation on their own is twofold. First, it gives them the opportunity
to talk about issues that concern them confidentially but it also introduces them
to the arrangement that they will come across when they move to an adult clinic
where it is likely that they will be expected to attend consultations alone.

> When they come to the adolescent clinic the emphasis is
> different in that we're concentrating on the child or the
> adolescent with input from the parent rather than what
> we're doing at the children's clinic which is involving the
> parent mainly with the child to some extent.
> *(Paediatric diabetes specialist nurse)*

However, there is flexibility in this arrangement so that young people also get
the opportunity to talk one to one with a team member.

> We know from a survey that we did that the patients like to
> see the doctor, so they do and the nurses usually see them
> with us but there is the option for them to go off elsewhere,
> and similarly with the dietician.
> *(Consultant paediatrician)*

The large caseload means that there is limited time allocated to each patient
although nurses and the dietician do offer to see young people between
appointments and do overrun the 15 minute appointment slot if it is felt necessary.

> Although the actual appointment time slots are very short
> and we don't usually keep to them, if somebody needs a
> longer time then they get a longer time, which is a good

thing for the family in the room but it's not such a
good thing for the family in the waiting room.
(Paediatric diabetes specialist nurse)

Screening

At every clinic, patients are weighed and measured and their blood measured
for HbA1c. HbA1c results are available immediately. They are asked to bring in
a urine sample for a microalbumen test, for renal function, although, as with all
clinics included in the study, staff reported that many teenagers fail to bring a
specimen with them. All those over 12 and who have had diabetes for four years
or more have retinal screening with their pupils dilated. They are also checked
for lipids, thyroid function and coeliac disease as part of the annual review.
Blood pressure is measured annually. Parents are asked to record the number of
hypos their children have experienced. Injection sites are also checked.

Location

The adolescent clinic is held in the hospital's outpatients department which staff
feel is not ideal because it is so busy. There is no dedicated unit for diabetes.

> It's basically a standard hospital outpatients and the waiting
> area isn't private, it's part of the corridor almost with people
> going back and forward to other clinic areas so that it's
> impossible to hold any kind of dialogue with parents or
> children there.
> *(Consultant paediatrician)*

The consulting rooms are not really large enough for the number of staff,
especially as family members are included in the consultation.

> As for the actual location and the environment, the way we
> do it is we work as a multidisciplinary team so we have
> everyone sitting in the room at the one time and it can get
> quite crowded like that if you have, you know, maybe three
> professionals in the room plus three family members. It can
> get quite cramped and the rooms aren't very large.
> *(Paediatric diabetes specialist nurse)*

Future plans

Although staff at the children's hospital feel that the current transition arrangements are not ideal, they cannot see how a smooth transition to adult care would be possible given that they refer to more than ten adult services. Most of the patients who attend the children's hospital live in the city but many are based outside it and some travel from outlying rural areas.

> I see transition to adult care as an area that is lacking.
> It would be much better if we could do that at a joint clinic
> but it's just physically not possible because we're transferring
> on to … It must be nigh on a dozen adult centres.
> *(Diabetes services coordinator)*

One suggestion is that diabetes services in the city could be reorganised so that fewer hospitals offer services to young people but that they are geographically located in, say, the north and south of the city. To achieve this, the services involved would have to agree which hospitals would provide services. If young people were transferred to only two, or perhaps three, adult services, it might be possible to offer transition clinics that were jointly staffed by paediatric and adult staff. Staff at the children's hospital are, however, already overstretched caring for their large and increasing caseload. Improved transition arrangements were, therefore, described by the consultant paediatrician as being 'on the agenda for discussion but a low priority' at the time of interview.

In all of the hospitals included in the study where clinics are held in outpatients departments, members of staff said they would prefer to be housed in a dedicated diabetes centre although the likelihood of this becoming a reality in any of the hospitals is not great at present.

> I would love a diabetes purpose built centre so that people
> could drop in, that we would have teaching areas, that we
> could also teach practice nurses, you know, GPs, student
> dieticians, student nurses, it would all be there and that's my
> desire. You know, an area specifically for the children and,
> you know, for different age groups of children because I
> think toddlers with diabetes need to be treated quite
> differently from school-aged children and, again, the
> adolescents are a group of their own too.
> *(Diabetes services coordinator)*

A less ambitious project is the production of a book for all patients and their families which is under way. Another is the development of a patient held record which each child or adolescent who attends the clinic will keep with details of their height, weight and glycaemic control. It is hoped that this will encourage young people to take an interest in their own care and become more involved in the process of monitoring their control.

> So that they hopefully will feel more ownership of the
> problem and not see it as us having to change things every
> four months, we want them to be able to see the reasons for
> changing it and act on their own initiative.
> *(Paediatrician)*

There is also a recently initiated programme of education targeted at adolescents who it is hoped will be responsive to learning more about diabetes. They have been offered the opportunity to meet with staff between clinics over a four-month period between routine clinics. They are invited to come to the hospital after school to learn more about diabetes, their treatment and the reasons for the screening that is undertaken with the aim of encouraging them to take more responsibility for their own care. The programme has been targeted at those whom staff deem it will most benefit because limited resources make it impossible to offer it to all patients but also because it is thought that some would not respond to the opportunity.

> What we try to do is to have them see that with small
> amounts of effort on their part and increased understanding
> that they actually can achieve improvements in their
> metabolic control. So that if we can guide them along for
> that four-month period, hopefully when they come back to
> clinic their control will be improved, and they will be able to
> say, 'Ah, I did that, that wasn't the diabetes team that did it
> for me'.
> *(Paediatrician)*

Research site F

The hospital is based in central London but accepts patients from a wide geographical area. It has a dedicated adolescent unit which includes both a ward for inpatients and outpatients' clinics.

The adolescent clinic

Hospital caseload size
119 patients aged 0–20

Ages of patients at transfer
Paediatric clinic ➔ Adolescent clinic: age 12
Adolescent clinic ➔ Adult clinic: age late teens or early 20s

Clinics
Frequency: 2 weeks out of 3
Time: 3.30 p.m.–6 p.m.
Number of patients per clinic: 8
Patients attend every 2 to 3 months
Location: Hospital adolescent unit

The diabetes team
Consultant paediatrician
Registrar
Paediatric diabetes specialist nurse
Paediatric dietician
Consultant clinical psychologist

Development of the adolescent service

The hospital houses a dedicated adolescent inpatient unit and the paediatrician who runs the diabetes service was employed to develop the service for adolescents in general. He specialises in diabetes and works only with adolescents.

The ages of young people

Young people join the adolescent clinic from the paediatric service based at a nearby children's hospital when they are around 12 years old and continue to attend until they are in their late teens or early twenties. The philosophy is that young people make the transition from the paediatric clinic to the adolescent clinic at about the same time as they transfer from primary to secondary school. There is no upper age limit in the adolescent clinic but the aim is to transfer patients to adult care from about the ages of 19 or 20. Recently some young people have remained in the adolescent service until after their twentieth birthday and this is in part because of plans to provide a young adult clinic in the near future.

Frequency, timing and size of the adolescent clinic

The adolescent diabetes clinic runs every two weeks between 3.30 p.m. and 6 p.m. At the time of the interviews, there were plans to run it every week because of caseload size. Appointments are more frequent than in the children's clinic so that staff can monitor glycaemic control during the period of adolescence when young people may find it difficult to manage diabetes.

> We like to see them more often than in paediatrics. We like to see them every two to three months because I think it is a time of dynamic change.
> *(Consultant paediatrician)*

Clinic structure

Young people are seen by staff alone and with their parents. They always have a consultation with the doctor and, in most cases, with the nurse too.

The staff team

The team includes the doctor, who is paediatrically trained but specialises in looking after adolescents, a diabetes specialist nurse, dietician and psychologist. There is also a registrar but the consultant, who believes continuity and consistency are important, ensures that he sees young people at least twice in every three appointments.

> They are learning to trust doctors, separately from their parents. And there is too much of this psychosocial stuff going on for them to see a different registrar every time they come and only to see the consultant once a year is pointless.
> *(Consultant paediatrician)*

Unlike most clinics, the adolescent service offers psychological support to all patients.

> We try and involve psychology in a normative sense which is saying that everybody with diabetes can have problems dealing with it. We'd like you all to know our psychologists and maybe meet them at different times when your diabetes is more problematic for you. It's not about seeing the psychologist if you're mad because everybody sees them. Most of the kids will buy that, not all of them.
> *(Consultant paediatrician)*

Staff were positive about the success of the multidisciplinary team where the specialist nurse has more responsibility than in the paediatric clinic and everyone's role is appreciated.

> I suppose we've developed over the last, say, three years, when we've worked together, a real shared sense of how we work which is a very open, patients-in-charge, solution focused approach.
> *(Consultant paediatrician)*

Screening

Young people are weighed and their height measured at all appointments. HbA1c is also measured and results are available immediately. There is an annual review where blood and urine are screened for liver and renal function, lipids, thyroid function and coeliac disease. Blood pressure is also measured and retinal screening carried out annually.

Location

The clinic is run in the adolescent unit so the location is dedicated to young people. There is an attractive waiting area with comfortable chairs, computers, music and a pool table. The teaching staff and youth worker who work with inpatients are available to talk to if necessary and the atmosphere is informal and friendly.

Future plans

As noted above, young people in their early twenties continue to attend the adolescent clinic. One of the reasons for this is that staff are in the process of developing a joint clinic with adult services for this age group. It is felt that young people should not move into a busy adult clinic where the majority of the other patients are both elderly and suffering from type 2 diabetes until they are at least 25. Like in the other hospitals included in the study, consultant time and space to run an additional clinic are scarce and improving services can be time-consuming and sometimes it is not possible to prioritise new developments because of existing workloads.

Other plans are to stratify the clinics further by age so that some clinics are for 13 to 16 year olds and others for older teenagers. Staff are also considering changing the structure of the clinic. They may offer activities supported by youth workers and teachers, allowing young people more choice about how they use their appointment and giving them more opportunities to make decisions about their care.

> I would like to develop some group work. I'd like to develop a system whereby kids come to clinic, clinic starts at 3.30 or whatever, but actually what we run is a fun, educational, bit of fun or whatever, beforehand, possibly for an hour which may be about the kids developing a website. And involve our youth workers and our teachers and all those people and have an ongoing, rolling, part educational but part recreational life skills programme as part of the clinic. Then they see us. What we'd like to develop is a system where they don't need to see me as the consultant each time. That they and us decide together – OK, you saw the doctor the last couple of times, we think you really need to see the dietician and actually you don't need to see anyone else this week.
> **(Consultant paediatrician)**

4.   The young people

The research sample

One of the aims of the research was to explore optimal procedures for
hand-over to adult care from the perspectives of young people with diabetes. A
central part of the study, therefore, was to interview young people who attend
the clinics in each research area. A sample of young people was identified in
each of the hospitals included in the study. In each research area, a member of
staff was asked to identify a cohort of young people who were in the year
approaching transfer to adult services and another cohort who had moved up
during the previous year. Because age of transfer differs across the sample
hospitals, the age group of the young people included was wide: the youngest at
first interview was ten years old and the oldest 24. The age at which young
people in areas B and D, for example, move into adult care is younger than in
areas C or F. The large majority of respondents was white and British.

Diabetes specialist nurses who had responsibility for caring for young people
wrote letters to potential respondents in each area giving details about the
research project and its aims and asking them if they would be willing to
participate as respondents. Those patients who were willing were then
approached by members of the research team.

The size of each research area's cohort was not the same because caseloads
varied between hospitals and because some potential respondents were
unwilling to participate or it proved impossible in the time scale available to
interview them. Young people were first interviewed between August 2000 and
April 2001 and again between August 2001 and April 2002.

Area cohorts also varied because of arrangements at different hospitals. The
cohort from area F, for example, did not include any respondents who had
moved out of adolescent care. The reason for this was that at the time of the

study, staff in area F were in the process of developing a clinic for young adults and the policy in the meantime was to retain young people in the care of the adolescent unit at the hospital. Conversely, there are only two respondents in the area D cohort who are still under the care of a paediatrician. The policy in area D is that adult diabetologists care for young people when they move into the adolescent clinic at the age of about 12 or 13. This meant that those still seeing paediatric staff were relatively young. In most cases, therefore, it was thought that the research instruments would not be suitable for their age group.

Although the large majority of young people invited to participate were willing to do so, a total of ten refused. The research team also faced difficulties in contacting some of those who were willing. Some were away at university, some had moved house or had changed their telephone numbers and failed to inform hospital staff and in some cases it was not possible to arrange a suitable time for an interview as potential respondents were working shifts and unable to plan ahead. A few had to be contacted a number of times as they had forgotten the interview appointment. In all, 16 young people who originally said they were willing to participate were not actually interviewed.

Although there were more young men (48) included in the study than young women (37), this was not because of any intended gender bias. Where individual hospital's caseloads were large, nurses at the hospitals selected an equal sample of both males and females but where there were fewer potential respondents it was not necessary to select and the complete cohort was included as potential respondents. The larger sample of young men does not imply that more young men than young women have diabetes.

The research design was longitudinal in the sense that the majority of young people were interviewed on two occasions. The second interview was carried out on the telephone. Those who had not yet moved out of paediatric care were interviewed in the year before they 'moved up' and then again approximately a year later. It was expected that these young people would have attended at least one appointment in the adult clinic by the time they were interviewed for the second time.

Of the 85 who were interviewed in the first round, 63 (74 per cent) participated in the second round of interviews. One would expect a certain level of attrition in any longitudinal study but perhaps particularly for a sample of this age group. Some young people could not be contacted a second time because they had either moved house or changed their telephone number without informing hospital staff. One was spending a year travelling abroad and another had died. Although others were contacted, it was not possible to interview them. In some cases, a number of arrangements were made to telephone them but they were always out or about to go out at the appointed time.

Of the 42 young people who were interviewed before they moved to adult care, 33 participated in the second round of interviews. Of these, 18 had moved from the clinic that they were attending at first interview, 13 continued to attend the same clinic and two did not know whether they had moved or not. Four of the 13 had had their final appointment at the clinic that they originally attended but had not yet been to their first adult appointment so were unable to comment on the differences.

Three groups of young people participated in the research study. First, there was the 'interview sample' who were interviewed and who also filled in a questionnaire about their quality of life. The second group, the 'questionnaire sample', filled in the quality of life questionnaire, and the third 'online sample' responded to an online questionnaire about their attitudes to diabetes clinics and their ideas for improving them. The following sections give background information about all these participants. All participants had type 1 diabetes.

The 'interview sample'

In all 85 young people were interviewed and completed a questionnaire. This group constituted the main sample which provided most of the data used in this report. They were recruited to the project because they attended one of the clinics in the six research areas (see Table 4.1).

Table 4.1 Numbers of young people in 'interview sample'

Research site	n	%
A	16	19
B	16	19
C	13	15
D	11	13
E	18	21
F	11	13
Total	85	100

Almost half of those who were interviewed were registered with some kind of transition diabetes service (see Figure 4.1), attending either an adolescent or a young adult clinic run jointly by staff from paediatric or adult services. The other half of the sample (43 individuals) attended an adult service and, of those, nine were attending an adolescent clinic run by adult physicians in research area D.

Figure 4.1 Clinic type

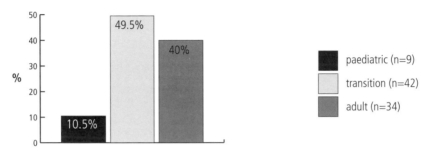

Young people were sampled by the type of clinic they were attending at the time of interview and not by age. The youngest participant was ten years old and the eldest was just 24 (mean age=17.6). The broad age range of respondents (see Figure 4.2) reflects the fact that the policies and practices of age banding clinics are widely variable in different diabetes services. In one hospital, for example, young people stop seeing a paediatrician at the age of 12 or 13 while, in another, young adults attend a jointly run clinic until they reach their early twenties.

Figure 4.2 Ages of respondents in the 'interview sample'

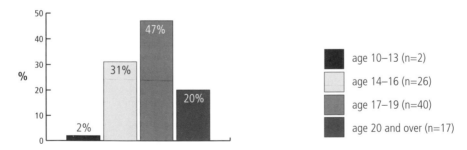

The ages at which young people in the 'interview sample' were diagnosed with diabetes varied from as young as one year to the oldest who was 15 (mean age=9 years) (see Figure 4.3).

Figure 4.3 Age at diagnosis of diabetes in the 'interview sample'

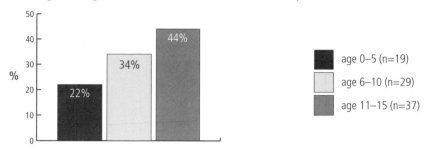

More males than females were interviewed (see Figure 4.4). In research areas where clinic caseloads were large enough, equal numbers of males and females were sampled but where all patients at a particular stage of transition to adult services were included it was not possible to balance numbers. No bias between males and females was intended when sampling.

Figure 4.4 Sex of respondents in the 'interview sample'

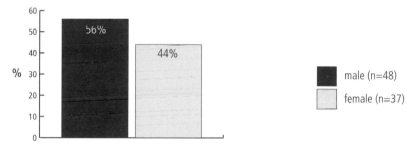

Two-thirds of 'interview sample' respondents were either at school or attended a college of further education, while a quarter were working or looking for work (Figure 4.5). Nearly three-quarters of the total were students at school, college or university.

Figure 4.5 Occupation of respondents in the 'interview sample'

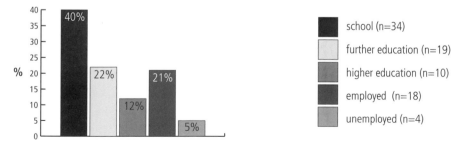

The large majority of young people (almost 90 per cent) in the 'interview sample' lived at home with their families (Figure 4.6). Those who had left home lived in shared accommodation, alone in a flat or, in one case, with a partner and young child.

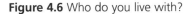
Figure 4.6 Who do you live with?

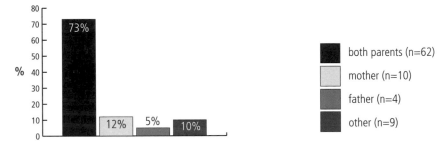

The 'questionnaire sample'

Young people who were interviewed were also asked, at the time of interview, to complete a quality of life questionnaire developed for teenagers with diabetes. A small number who did not have time returned the questionnaire by post after the interview and a total of 78 questionnaires were completed by the original sample of 85. All those who were interviewed for a second time were sent another copy of the questionnaire and asked to complete and return it. Despite reminder telephone calls, only 44 (70 per cent) of the 63 respondents who were interviewed on two occasions returned the questionnaire. An analysis of the data collected from the quality of life questionnaires can be found in Chapter 10.

This quality of life measure had not been validated previously because a large enough sample was not available at the time of its development. Research staff at the National Children's Bureau collaborated with psychologists at Royal Holloway, University of London, in order to increase the current project's sample size of 78 to make it large enough for the necessary psychometric testing to be carried out for the purpose of validation. This larger sample has been called the 'questionnaire sample'. Questionnaires were sent, or handed out at clinic appointments, to an extra 204 young people aged 13 to 17 who were identified by nurses at five of the hospitals included in the study. Staff at the sixth hospital were undertaking another research study with adolescents in their care and so were unwilling to increase the sample as they were concerned that patients could become 'research weary'. An extra 80 respondents (51 per cent of the total sample) completed the questionnaire, making the overall 'questionnaire sample' who filled in the quality of life measure 158 (see Table 4.2).

Table 4.2 Completed questionnaires by research site

Research site	n	%
A	30	19
B	46	29
C	26	17
D	25	16
E	21	13
F	10	6
Total	158	100

The response rate for those who completed the quality of life measure but who did not participate in interviews was greater from females (25 per cent) than from males (15 per cent). Fifty were female and 30 male. Young people who attended four of the hospitals were sent a copy of the questionnaire to their homes with a covering letter and the overall response rate from these hospitals was 49 per cent (76 out of a sample of 154). At one hospital the questionnaires were not posted but given to young people when they attended clinic appointments (with a covering letter). The response rate from this hospital was very low: only four questionnaires were received back out of 50 distributed. All young people were sent or given a freepost envelope in which to return the questionnaire. The covering letter explained the purpose of the questionnaire and that respondents' anonymity would be preserved.

The additional respondents included in the 'questionnaire sample' were not asked what kind of clinic they attended but none had yet transferred to adult care. They either attended an adolescent clinic run by a paediatric department or a clinic jointly run by paediatric and adult staff. They were not asked who they lived with although it can be assumed that the large majority of the 80 respondents who were not interviewed and who were all aged between 11 and 17 had not yet left home.

The mean age of the 'questionnaire sample' was younger than that of the 'interview sample' (16.3 years compared with 17.6 years), with over half aged between 14 and 16 years (Figure 4.7).

Figure 4.7 Ages of respondents in the 'questionnaire sample'

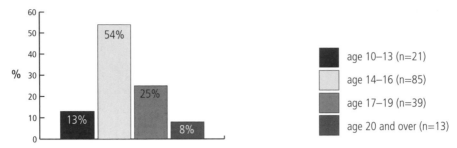

Like those in the 'interview sample', these respondents were more likely to have been diagnosed with diabetes over the age of 11 than at a younger age (Figure 4.8). Less than a quarter had been diagnosed under the age of six.

Figure 4.8 Age at diagnosis of diabetes in the 'questionnaire sample'

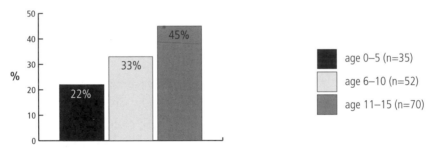

One respondent did not give their age at diagnosis

In contrast to the 'interview sample', the majority of the 'questionnaire sample' was female (Figure 4.9). Although questionnaires were sent to equal numbers of males and females, more females responded.

Figure 4.9 Sex of respondents in the 'questionnaire sample'

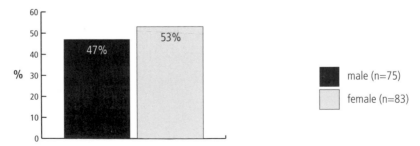

In line with their younger age profile, nearly two-thirds (63 per cent) of respondents in the 'questionnaire sample' were at school and over three-quarters (78 per cent) at school or attending sixth form college (Figure 4.10). Of the whole sample, 85 per cent were studying at school, college or in higher education.

Figure 4.10 Occupation of respondents in the 'questionnaire sample'

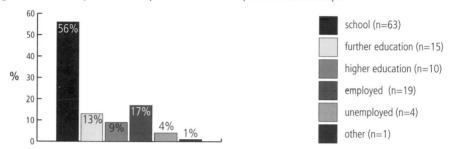

The online sample
==================

In order to increase the size and diversity of the sample of young people with diabetes, it was agreed to post an online questionnaire on the Diabetes Explained website (www.diabetes-explained.co.uk). This site is aimed at young people with diabetes and offers general information on living with diabetes and a message board where visitors to the site can post questions or observations. The aim of using an online questionnaire was to find out what respondents felt about attending clinic appointments. It included questions specifically about likes and dislikes and how health services could be improved to suit respondents' needs. The invitation to respond was open to all young visitors to the site who were willing to complete the questionnaire and focused on clinic attendance and how users of hospital services felt about their quality, accessibility and appropriateness. The large majority of those who completed the questionnaire described themselves as 'good attenders' or 'pretty good attenders' of clinic appointments (30 individuals) while only four ticked 'awful attender – I hardly ever go'. Responses were anonymous so hospitals attended by respondents are unknown. Fifty-one questionnaires were completed and findings are reported in Chapter 5.

Inviting visitors to a website to participate in a survey is, of course, a relatively new opportunity for researchers. An online survey offers respondents the chance to give their opinions anonymously but it is not possible for researchers to verify their details (Ó Dochartaigh 2002). The young people who completed the online questionnaire may not, in fact, be young and may not have diabetes and it must therefore be acknowledged that all data from this source may not be valid although responses to questions about diabetes clinics make it seem unlikely that respondents were not genuine. However, the internet is a useful tool for making contact with large numbers of potential research respondents, particularly those who may be traditionally hard to reach, and the research team felt that results from the online survey were a useful addition to data collected by more traditional methods.

Of the 51 young people who responded to the online questionnaire, 41 (80 per cent) reported that they were registered with a clinic, seven that they were not and three did not respond to this question. However, all 51 answered a question about what kind of clinic they attended (Figure 4.11). Just over half of the online respondents (53 per cent) were registered with either a children's or adolescent clinic, while the rest attended adult services. Five individuals were not sure what kind of clinic they attended.

Figure 4.11 Clinic type attended by respondents in the 'online sample'

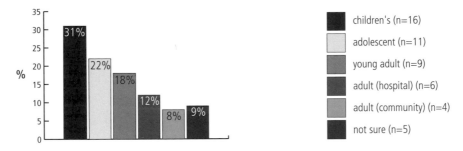

Nearly 70 per cent of the online sample were aged between 14 and 19 and there were only six under 14 (Figure 4.12). The youngest was ten and the oldest 24 years old. They were not asked their age at diagnosis of diabetes.

Figure 4.12 Ages of respondents in the 'online sample'

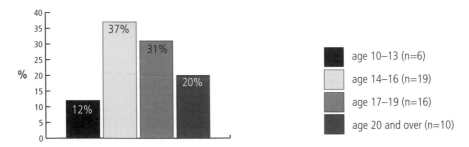

There were more than three times the number of female respondents than male (Figure 4.13). Like those who returned the quality of life questionnaires, it seems that young women are more likely than young men to respond to questionnaires.

Figure 4.13 Sex of respondents in the 'online sample'

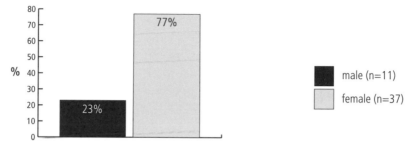

Three respondents did not give their gender.

Non-attenders of clinic appointments

Young people with diabetes may lose contact with medical services at the point when they are taking increasing responsibility for their own condition and in the process of being transferred from paediatric to adult care (Kipps *et al.* 2002). There may be a number of reasons why young people stop attending clinic appointments at this time. They may move away from home, parents may stop taking responsibility for their attendance and accompanying them to the clinic or 'adult sub-speciality clinics may have a less individual, holistic and family-centred approach than has previously been experienced' (Kurtz *et al.* 1996).

One of the aims of the study was to elicit reasons why some young people fail to keep in contact with services. Although just over half (54 per cent) of the young people in the interview sample reported having missed at least one clinic appointment, only one was a persistent non-attender. Although it is not uncommon for adult patients who fail to attend two consecutive appointments to be removed from case lists, paediatric staff, particularly diabetes specialist nurses, make a concerted effort to keep in contact with young people with diabetes and encourage them to attend appointments.

It was hoped that the sample would include a cohort of young people in each area who had failed to attend at least two consecutive clinic appointments in order to explore the reasons why some young people are unwilling to access health services. Because of the difficulty in identifying such a cohort in any of the areas included in the study, it was not possible to include a meaningful sample. However, insights into why young people may not make use of services are included in the analysis of data collected (see Chapter 5). Despite the study's specified aim of exploring the reasons why some young people fail to attend hospital appointments, it was not possible to identify a group who persistently reject medical services. The sample was selected through the auspices of hospital staff who try to ensure that contact is maintained with patients even if some appointments are missed. If further research aims to explore the question of non-attendance at appointments amongst this group, another sampling technique should perhaps be investigated.

Interviews with young people

For the first round of interviews most young respondents were interviewed face to face in their homes although, for their own preference and/or convenience, five met the interviewer in pubs or cafés. Most interviews were undertaken one to one but, in some cases, a parent or sibling was present. Interviews in the first round took about an hour to complete. Interviews in the second round were carried out by telephone at a time agreed beforehand by each young person and were shorter in length. Second round interviews were carried out approximately a year after the first round.

A draft interview schedule was piloted with three young people who were not included in the study. It became clear from this piloting exercise that the interview schedules should be semi-structured and include both closed and open questions. This was to ensure that sufficient data was collected from those respondents who were shy or felt they had little to say about their care as well as those who were more eloquent. All interviews were tape recorded (except where this was not possible because of background noise) with the respondent's consent.

The interviews elicited both quantitative (such as age of diagnosis and regularity of clinic appointments) and qualitative data covering respondents' experiences of and feelings about diabetes care. Subjects included were how young people perceived the clinic environment, the timing of clinics, relationships with staff and the move from children's to adult services. Feelings about missed appointments, the availability of support from hospital staff between appointments and the use of GP services were also discussed. Respondents were also invited to share their aspirations for an ideal transition which included the optimal age for 'moving up', the preferred setting for young people's services, the timing of clinics and the facilities they would like available.

Tape recorded interviews were transcribed and analysed using the NVivo program. Quantitative data was entered into a database in SPSS (Statistical Package for Social Sciences) for analysis.

Ethical considerations

Interviews with young people and staff were undertaken in strictest confidence and all respondents were assured of anonymity and confidentiality of personal information as indicated by the Data Protection Act. Approval for the study was sought from and agreed by the London Multicentre Research Ethics Committee as well as eight Local Research Ethics Committees. Young people were asked to provide written consent before participating and were given the opportunity to opt out of the study at any time. No inpatients were included.

5. Attendance and non-attendance at clinic appointments

Going to the clinic

Young people who participated in the research interviews were asked about their attendance at the diabetes clinic, whether it was easy to travel to clinic appointments and whether attendance interfered with their other activities. Regular clinic appointments when blood glucose levels can be measured and adjustments made to insulin dose are a vital component of diabetes care and it is important therefore that services are easily accessible for young people. This chapter also focuses on non-attendance at diabetes clinics and the reasons why some young people fail to go to appointments.

Frequency of appointments

Almost all of the 85 young people included in the study attended clinic appointments at least every six months (98 per cent) although nearly half attended every three months or more often (46 per cent). A small number reported that they saw a diabetes specialist nurse between clinic appointments if, for example, they had recently changed their insulin dose or had particular problems with maintaining a diet or had high blood glucose levels. A third of those who had not yet moved to an adult clinic reported that the frequency of appointments had remained the same over recent years while 40 per cent reported that their appointments were less frequent than they had been previously. Three individuals said that clinic frequency varied depending on their blood glucose control or current regimen. Of the 42 who had moved into adult care, 70 per cent were attending less frequently than they had previously in transition or paediatric clinics.

Getting to the clinic

Although there was only one young person in the sample who had persistently failed to attend hospital appointments, the study focused on access to services for all young people. Respondents were asked about how they travelled to the clinic, how long it took to get there and whether attending appointments interfered with their education or employment.

Over 90 per cent of respondents reported that getting to the clinic was 'very easy' or 'quite easy' (Table 5.1). A minority, particularly those living in rural areas, had to travel a long way to the clinic and so found it more difficult to get there. However, over 90 per cent said they could travel to the clinic in less than an hour (Table 5.2). The one young person who reported that it was 'very difficult' to travel to the clinic had to travel by air!

Table 5.1 How easy is it to get to the clinic?

	n	%
Very easy	42	50
Quite easy	35	41
Quite difficult	7	8
Very difficult	1	1
Total	85	100

Table 5.2 How long does it take to get to the clinic?

	n	%
Less than half an hour	54	63
Half an hour or more	26	31
An hour or more	4	5
Two hours or more	1	1
Total	85	100

The majority (61 per cent) travelled to the clinic by car and almost all of these were driven by a parent. Over a quarter travelled by public transport while the others walked or cycled to the clinic.

Timing of clinics

Although health care staff in some hospitals have tried to fit clinics around young people's schedules in order to encourage them to attend, the majority of clinics run during the working day (Table 5.3). There were no weekend clinics. There was little difference in timing of paediatric, transition or adult clinics.

Table 5.3 When are your clinic appointments?

	Before transfer		After transfer		Total	
	n	%	n	%	n	%
During school/work hours	25	60	27	63	52	61
After school/work hours	14	33	15	35	29	34
During school or university holidays	3	7	1	2	4	5
Total	42	100	43	100	85	100

However, just under half said that attending clinics did not interfere with their work 'at all' (Table 5.4). In fact, some young people viewed daytime clinics positively as they meant a morning or afternoon off school. A greater proportion of those who attended adult clinics said that clinic attendance affected their education 'a bit' or 'not much'.

Table 5.4 Do clinic appointments interfere with school/college/work?

	Before transfer		After transfer		Total	
	n	%	n	%	n	%
Yes, a lot	4	10	4	10	8	10
Yes, a bit	4	10	8	19	12	14
Not much	7	16	15	36	22	26
Not at all	27	64	14	33	41	49
Don't know			1	2	1	1
Total	42	100	42	100	84	100

One 'after transfer' respondent did not answer this question

What's the clinic like?

Young people were asked about the clinic's environment and atmosphere. The large majority found the clinic they attended welcoming and friendly and only very few thought it depressing or intimidating (Table 5.5).

Table 5.5 Atmosphere at clinics

Is the clinic...	welcoming?		depressing?		friendly?		scary?	
	n	%	n	%	n	%	n	%
Yes, very	43	50	3	4	44	52		
Yes, quite	27	32	4	5	33	39	4	5
Not very	9	11	8	9	5	6	6	7
No	4	5	68	80	1	1	73	86
Don't know	2	2	2	2	2	2	2	2
Total	85	100	85	100	85	100	85	100

A majority of all those interviewed found the clinics clean, comfortable, spacious, modern and easy to find (Table 5.6), although a number said that it had been difficult to find on their first visit.

Table 5.6 Clinic environment

Is the clinic...	clean?		comfortable?		spacious?		modern?		easy to find?	
	n	%	n	%	n	%	n	%	n	%
Yes, very	50	59	23	27	18	21	16	19	33	39
Yes, quite	32	38	52	61	39	46	31	36	37	43
Not very	1	1	7	8	24	28	22	26	8	10
Not at all			2	3	3	4	12	14	6	7
Don't know	2	2	1	1	1	1	4	5	1	1
Total	85	100	85	100	85	100	85	100	85	100

On the whole they were not critical of clinic facilities although 40 per cent thought the environment might be improved to suit their age group and over 60 per cent felt that there should be more to do in the waiting room (Table 5.7).

Table 5.7 Are there ways that the clinic could improve for people of your age?

	Environment		Waiting times		Things to do while waiting	
	n	%	n	%	n	%
Definitely	17	20	17	20	33	39
Maybe	17	20	13	16	19	23
Probably not	35	42	39	46	24	28
Not at all	15	18	15	18	8	10
Total	84	100	84	100	84	100

One person did not answer this question

More than half said there was a shop or café in the hospital where they could get something to eat or drink (Table 5.8). Two hospitals had facilities for making tea and coffee in the clinic which were available to patients and their families.

Table 5.8 Availability of food and drinks at the clinic

Is there a…	cold drinks machine in the clinic?		hot drinks machine in the clinic?		café in the hospital?		shop in the hospital?		other facility in the hospital?	
	n	%	n	%	n	%	n	%	n	%
Yes	22	26	24	28	49	58	49	58	3	3
No	54	63	52	61	26	30	26	30	73	86
Don't know	9	11	9	11	10	12	10	12	9	11
Total	85	100	85	100	85	100	85	100	85	100

The majority (88 per cent) said they never or rarely had to wait to be seen (Table 5.9) although over 60 per cent described the clinic as 'very' or 'quite' busy.

Table 5.9 Being seen on time

	n	%
Always on time	41	48
Usually on time	34	40
Often later	7	8
Always later	1	1
Don't know	2	3
Total	85	100

More than 90 per cent of young people felt they 'always' or 'usually' had enough time to talk to staff at clinic appointments (Table 5.10).

Table 5.10 Is there enough time to talk to health care staff at the clinic?

	n	%
Yes, always	56	67
Yes, usually	20	24
Yes, sometimes	5	6
No	3	3
Total	84	100

One person did not answer this question

The 43 young people who had moved from paediatric to adult care were also asked to compare their experience of attending both clinics (Table 5.11). Over 90 per cent found the location of the adult clinic more convenient or 'about the same' as the one they had attended previously. The large majority also found appointment times (83 per cent) and the frequency of appointments (95 per cent) more convenient or 'about the same'.

Table 5.11 Comparison of adult clinic with previous clinic

	Location		Appointment times		Frequency of appointments	
	n	%	n	%	n	%
More convenient	13	29	5	12	13	29
About the same	27	64	31	71	28	66
Less convenient	3	7	5	12		
Don't know			2	5	2	5
Total	43	100	43	100	43	100

Contact with staff at the clinic

Young people were most likely to see a doctor (100 per cent) and diabetes specialist nurse (DSN) (92 per cent) at clinic appointments (Table 5.12). Although more than half (52 per cent) reported that they had contact with a dietician, 44 per cent said they never received specialist dietetic advice. Thirty-five young people (41 per cent of the sample) had their eyes checked regularly outside the clinic. Five individuals also reported that they had seen a podiatrist outside the clinic. Medical complications of diabetes are associated with the duration of the condition as well as glycaemic control and therefore young people may only be seen by an optometrist or a podiatrist, who screen for the early onset of complications, if they have had diabetes for a certain length of time. Endocrinologists looking after young people with diabetes are also trained to check eyes and feet for signs of retinopathy and neuropathy.

The three respondents who had had contact with a psychologist attended the hospital in research area F where clinical psychologists are part of the multidisciplinary team.

Table 5.12 How often do you see health care staff at clinic?

	Doctor		DSN		Dietician	
	n	%	n	%	n	%
Every three months	33	39	34	41	8	9
At least twice a year	42	50	31	37	11	13
At least once a year	5	6	6	7	9	11
Other	4	5	2	2	16	19
Don't know			4	5	3	4
Never			7	8	37	44
Total	84	100	84	100	84	100

One respondent had not attended a clinic appointment for some time and did not respond

Although the majority of young people travelled to the clinic with a parent, more than half consulted with the doctor and nurse on their own. In some cases, the young person went into the consultation alone and then their parent was invited to join them.

Table 5.13 Do you see health care staff alone or with someone else?

	Doctor		DSN	
	n	%	n	%
Alone	42	51	44	57
With a parent	26	31	18	23
Alone and with a parent	12	15	12	16
With someone else	1	1	1	1
It varies	2	2	2	3
Total	83[1]	100	77[2]	100

1 One respondent had not attended a clinic appointment for some time and did not answer this question. One respondent did not see a doctor at her first appointment in the adult clinic and did not answer this question.
2 Eight respondents did not regularly see a nurse and did not answer this question.

Diabetes care between appointments

An important aspect of diabetes care is the availability of advice and support between appointments. Young people or their parents may occasionally need urgent advice, particularly regarding illness, but may also sometimes want reassurance or information. Young people were asked about whether they had ever contacted members of staff between appointments and, if so, how easy it was to gain access to a member of staff. Patients or their parents were much more likely to contact a diabetes specialist nurse than a doctor (Table 5.14).

Table 5.14 Contacting a member of staff

	Doctor		DSN	
	n	%	n	%
Yes, quite often	1	1	5	6
Yes, occasionally	5	6	36	43
Yes, once	5	6	7	8
No	73	87	36	43
Total	84	100	84	100

One respondent did not answer this question

Of those 55 respondents who had tried to contact a member of staff by telephone, nearly 60 per cent had found that they could 'always' or 'usually' get in touch easily (Table 5.15). However, 35 per cent said it was not easy to make contact.

Table 5.15 Contacting a member of staff by phone

	n	%
Yes, always easy	20	36
Yes, usually easy	12	22
Yes, sometimes easy	4	7
Not easy	19	35
Total	55	100

One respondent described how it can be difficult to track down a specialist nurse.

> It's good but like if you do need the nurse and you are
> trying to get hold of them, sometimes it can be really easy
> and sometimes you might get passed from person to person
> because they are not quite sure. It can be a bit confusing

and difficult at times but, if you manage to get hold of them, then they are there for you.

(18 year old female)

Many diabetes specialist nurses who work with children make home visits, particularly in the period immediately after diagnosis. Over half (55 per cent) of respondents had been visited at home more than once by a nurse and two-thirds at least once (Table 5.16). In some areas, nurses are able to meet with adolescents at home too although geographical location and caseload size are factors in making this possible or not. Both nurses and young people felt that the quality of these consultations was enhanced by the informal setting. Meeting young people in their own homes also allowed nurses to get to know them and their families better and this helped them tailor their advice to a young person's particular circumstances.

Working as I do, going into their homes, you get to know them very well and you see the other bits to their lives that you don't see in a clinic setting. I feel that that improves the relationship really because you're looking at them holistically if you like as opposed to just a diabetic who's of such and such an age. You can actually use that information and bring it into the clinic and improve things here.

(Paediatric diabetes specialist nurse)

We need more DSNs [diabetes specialist nurses] who are out there, seeing kids in their homes. Time after time we are seeing kids with poor control and we talk to them, do their education but it's so different if you go into someone's house and you actually sit down with them at their kitchen table. You look at what they are eating and you look at the way they are injecting, and you look at the way the house is running.

(Consultant paediatrician)

Table 5.16 Has a nurse visited you at home?

	n	%
Yes, more than once	47	55
Yes, once	10	12
No	27	32
Don't remember	1	1
Total	85	100

It became clear from talking to young people that some nurses make a special effort to see young people at home or to contact them by telephone and, in some cases, make their own home telephone number available.

> That's when I would phone [the nurse] at home [i.e. out of hospital hours] because she has always said that that's alright, but I don't make a habit of it. I just know if it's really bad then she is there.
> *(17 year old female)*

> I think it is good because if I don't get in contact with them they will always ring up at home to see how I am. They are always making sure.
> *(17 year old male)*

> They're approachable, they know what they're talking about, they give advice but they don't ram it down your throat. You can make appointments to see them outside the clinic.
> *(18 year old male)*

> Her auntie lives across the road so when she goes to pick up her little boy she will pop in if I have any problems. She knows I'll be here then.
> *(17 year old female)*

Most young people were satisfied with their experience of attending diabetes clinics and with the care available between appointments. Most could travel easily to the clinic from home, school or work and, despite the fact that the majority of clinics were held during the working day, attendance did not have an adverse effect on education or on working lives. Most young people reported that they did not have to wait to be seen by clinic staff. Participants in the study were also, in the main, happy with the clinic environment and atmosphere although they would like to have more magazines and relevant literature or a television in the waiting room.

More than half of those young people who had telephoned a nurse between clinic appointments had been able to make contact but over a third had found it difficult to get through to the person they wanted to speak to. Home visits by nurses were appreciated by young people who felt the informal contact gave them an opportunity to get to know nurses better and to talk more freely about all aspects of living with diabetes.

A large proportion of the young people interviewed had not consulted a dietician for some time. Although all those interviewed (who attended clinic appointments) reported that they saw a doctor at least once a year, only 22 per cent said they saw a dietician at least every six months and 44 per cent said they never saw a dietician. Only three individuals had had contact with a psychologist and these all attended one hospital where psychological services are readily available. Respondents to a survey of paediatricians caring for young people with diabetes carried out in 1998 under the auspices of Diabetes UK (Jefferson *et al.* 2003) reported that dieticians attended 86 per cent of paediatric clinics and over half (55 per cent) reported that their diabetes clinic had easy access to a podiatrist. Just over a quarter of respondents to the same survey reported that a 'counsellor' regularly attended children's diabetes clinics. Most of these were psychologists, with some clinics supported by a psychiatrist or a nurse therapist. The findings from this study suggest that some young people are not getting access to regular dietetic advice and that the large majority do not have immediate access to psychological services. The evidence is as reported by young people and it may be, however, that dietetic advice is available but that young people are either not aware of it or are unwilling to take advantage of it.

Online participants and attendance at clinic appointments

As noted in Chapter 4, a supplementary sample of 51 young people participated in the study by giving their views on diabetes care in a questionnaire posted on an internet website. The reason for recruiting extra respondents was to include an anonymous sample of young people who might not have been regular clinic attenders as this group was under-represented in the main sample. The responses were sent electronically to the Diabetes Explained website (www.diabetes-explained.co.uk) between April 2001 and June 2002.

Although two-thirds of respondents reported that they 'like' or 'don't mind' attending clinic appointments, 29 per cent said they hated going (Figure 5.1). However, the large majority (over 75 per cent) described themselves as 'good attenders' who always go to clinic (Figure 5.2) and very few, only four individuals, described themselves as 'awful' attenders who rarely go to appointments.

Figure 5.1 How do you feel about going to clinic appointments?

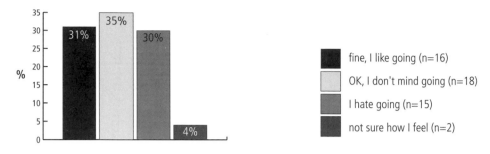

fine, I like going (n=16)

OK, I don't mind going (n=18)

I hate going (n=15)

not sure how I feel (n=2)

Figure 5.2 Attending appointments

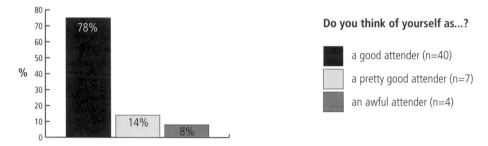

Do you think of yourself as...?

a good attender (n=40)

a pretty good attender (n=7)

an awful attender (n=4)

It is encouraging that so many of those who responded to the online questionnaire attend clinic appointments regularly, even though some do not enjoy the experience. Perhaps it should be expected that young people who are interested enough in diabetes to log on to a diabetes education website are also likely to be clinic attenders. However, hospital staff should consider why some young people 'hate' going to clinic appointments.

The majority of those who added comments to their responses were positive about the diabetes service and, particularly, about their relationships with staff, although there were some dissenters. Five were glad to get time off school or work in order to attend appointments while three said that they did not want to miss school or work. In terms of changes that could be made to improve the experience of going to the clinic, long waiting times were mentioned most often (by six respondents). Other comments focused on the way respondents feel they are treated by staff and their desire for autonomy and understanding. For example:

> [The clinic should be] a place where the advice was neutral
> and where the doctors and nurses don't hide facts.
> *(24 year old male)*

Not patronising.
(15 year old female)

Do things when I am ready for them (in my time).
(16 year old female)

I'd like to be treated like an adult that knows what she is
doing.
(17 year old female)

If they understood that at our age you feel like you want to
live the same life as any other person.
(19 year old female)

Other suggestions were for age banded clinics arranged in such a way that
young people would have the opportunity to talk to each other, and better
information resources.

Non-attendance at clinic appointments

Providers of diabetes services are concerned about young people's non-
attendance at outpatient clinic appointments, which may become more
common at the point of transfer to adult services (Kipps *et al.* 2002). The
physiological effects of puberty and growth, changing lifestyles and increased
responsibility for self-care all mean that maintaining optimal glycaemic control
can be more difficult during adolescence. Regular contact with the diabetes
team is important in order to monitor blood glucose levels, provide information
to the young person and, if appropriate, alter the individual's treatment to allow
a more appropriate approach to maximising glycaemic control. In order to
encourage attendance, clinics should be accessible and acceptable to young
people and there should be procedures to ensure that young people are
followed up if they fail to keep in contact with services. Guidelines on the care
of young people, for example, suggest the diabetes team should ensure that
'there is no hiatus in care at the time of transfer and that the young person is
not lost to follow-up care' (ISPAD 2000).

Some young people, however, do fail to attend clinic appointments and may lose
touch with services altogether. This may come at a time when glycaemic control is
difficult to attain and may, in the longer term, be a factor in the development of
medical complications. There is evidence that there is a higher incidence of such

complications amongst those who do not attend clinic appointments. For young people diagnosed with diabetes in early childhood, the risks may be particularly high as they will be particularly susceptible to complications because of the length of time they have been living with the condition.

> Young people with diabetes who are lost to follow-up care
> have a high risk of vascular complications.
> *(ISPAD 2000)*

> Regular attendance maximises the opportunity of stabilising
> their condition and achieving the metabolic control
> necessary to reduce the risk of long-term complications.
> *(Wilson and Greenhalgh 1999)*

Guidelines for managing diabetes in children and young adults produced by ISPAD (2000) identify 'failure of attendance at clinics particularly at the time of transition from paediatric to adult services' as a major risk and recommend that services 'should have mechanisms in place to identify and locate all young people who fail to attend follow-up consultations'. It is important that procedures for the transition to adult care are clear to young people and their families in order to minimise non-attendance and that young adults newly referred to adult services are not discouraged from keeping appointments. In the interviews, young people were asked about their preferences for transition arrangements. The majority were in favour of being transferred to a young adult clinic where staff have an expertise in providing services to this age group.

Staff who were interviewed confirmed that attendance at young people's clinics can be poor. Data collected from clinics on non-attendance at particular clinics was variable but at least one person booked for a clinic failed to attend in all areas where data was returned and on all occasions. The Audit Commission's report, *Testing times* (2000) identified non-attendance as a particular problem in young adults and this was confirmed by a consultant who runs a young person's clinic who said:

> The most common default clinic is a young persons' clinic. The
> default is about 20 per cent of the routine clinics and there
> might be 30 per cent at the young persons' clinic. One of the
> reasons we moved from an 'adolescent' clinic to a 'young
> adults' clinic was that we were sitting twiddling our thumbs
> because more than half of the people didn't turn up to it.
> *(Consultant diabetologist – adult service)*

One of the aims of the research was to explore the extent to which young people in the sample failed to attend services and the reasons they gave for not turning up for clinic appointments. As noted above, there was only one persistent non-attender in the sample but questions about clinic attendance were included in interviews with both young people and medical staff. Additional responses about the issue of attendance at clinic were received from young people who logged on to the Diabetes Explained website. Diabetes team members at each research site were also asked about clinic attendance. Although staff reported that some young people did fail to attend, sometimes they themselves did not know why:

> We really don't know about why people don't come.
> *(Consultant diabetologist – adult service)*

One paediatric nurse described a variety of reasons why she thought young patients and their families failed to attend.

> Sometimes it can be that there's a problem developed in the family unrelated to diabetes, a marriage break-up or something like that that's causing a lot of stress. Sometimes it can be rebellion in the actual child themselves and the child if it's a teenager point blankly refuses to come. Sometimes it can be that the parent may not have liked either an approach or a person, something like that. There may have been something in the clinic that the parent hasn't liked and they're trying to avoid that. Sometimes it's just that the families, if they live quite an erratic lifestyle, can literally just keep forgetting and sometimes it can be that they move house a few times and we just don't know where they are.
> *(Paediatric diabetes specialist nurse)*

A 'core' (as staff described them) of young people persistently default from clinic attendance even when reminded by clinic staff but on the whole non-attendance is less deliberate and most young people come to at least half the appointments they are booked for. Staff did not necessarily expect more from this age group.

> I'm just pleased if they turn up for two out of the four [adolescent] clinics in the year. I think the adult team have got different expectations because they would expect adults to be responsible and turn up for their clinic appointment,

> full stop. Whereas I just think of them as, well, as I say, I'm
> pleased if they turn up for two out of the four. I think
> they're doing OK if that happens.
> *(Paediatric diabetes specialist nurse)*

Another nurse agreed that young people cannot be expected to behave like adults:

> I would do everything possible to make that appointment as
> pleasant and easy for them as possible because some contact
> is better than none and I don't subscribe to the theory that
> it's their responsibility, let them get on with it.
> *(Paediatric diabetes specialist nurse)*

Apart from the potential risks to young people with diabetes of failing to have their condition regularly monitored, non-attendance is also a cost to the health service. Patient non-attendance 'makes clinics inefficient … and wastes clerical and perhaps medical resources' (Simmons *et al.* 1997) and it is in the best interests of health care staff to identify whether particular groups of patients are less likely to attend and to develop strategies to reduce non-attendance. A number of hospitals have already carried out such audits (Dyer *et al.* 1998, Watson and Forshaw 2002). Evidence from existing audits shows that there is a wide variation in default rates but that social deprivation, which might mean not owning a car or a telephone, for example, is a factor. One study (Watson and Forshaw 2002) found that a third of paediatric patients who did not attend appointments were known to social services. Griffin (1998) argues that there are many factors that might predispose particular patients to non-attendance including patients' health beliefs, relationships with clinic staff, the way the clinic is organised, the level and extent of patient participation within consultations and the financial costs of attendance.

Why do some young people fail to attend?

Of the sample of 85 young people, 68 per cent said they always attend regularly, 26 per cent said they usually attend regularly and 6 per cent said they did not attend regularly. However, over half (55 per cent) had failed to attend at least one clinic appointment and, of these, the most common reason was 'I forgot' (32 per cent). Other reasons given for non-attendance were that the clinic was at an inconvenient time, they had another commitment or were on holiday or unwell. The large majority (84 per cent)of those who had failed to attend an appointment said that they did not mind having missed it.

Although most young people did turn up regularly for clinic appointments, one explained the reasons why he would prefer not to go:

> Things I don't like about the clinic is the actual fact of going there. It would be a lot easier if someone came to you. It takes up your time. There was a lot of course work in school and there'll be a lot of college work, so it takes up your time going there.
> *(15 year old male)*

For some, going to the clinic is an unpleasant chore they would rather not have to do even though they acknowledge its usefulness:

> They're helpful but personally I don't like hospitals at all.
> *(18 year old male)*

> It's a bit of a drag. As soon as I'm there I just want to get home. It's a good place but I can't be bothered with it.
> *(16 year old male)*

> I don't really have any feelings one way or the other. Going to clinics is like school – it's a drag but you have to go and it's for the better so you live with it.
> *(14 year old male)*

> I don't like going 'cause I don't wanna find out if it's getting any worse. I get really nervous before I go. The only good thing about going is that I can ask a few questions. It's also good 'cause we can get our HbA1c result while we are waiting to see the doctor.
> *(16 year old female)*

It was not possible to collect clear evidence of why some young people persistently fail to attend appointments while others occasionally miss appointments but continue to go fairly regularly, if reluctantly. However, both young people and diabetes team members identified reasons why going to the clinic might be an uncomfortable experience.

'I forgot'

As noted above, the most common reason for non-attendance at a clinic appointment amongst the young people included in the study was that they had simply forgotten about it. In the experience of the researchers, clinic appointments are not the only engagements young people forget: a number also forgot about interviews that had been booked in advance and were either out or asleep when the researcher called to talk to them! One of the reasons for forgetting is that appointments are spaced out by months, or up to a year in the adult clinic, and there is often no reminder mechanism so that a busy, absent-minded teenager may have good reason to forget about it.

> If it's not for another year the card gets filed away somewhere and then that's it, it's gone! Whereas when it was in the child's clinic it was every three or four months so it was easier to remember.
> *(21 year old male)*

At the point at which young people are taking more responsibility for themselves, forgetting occasionally may be inevitable. There may be a period when they still expect to be reminded by a parent. One university student who lives away from home admitted:

> I think I've been relying on my mum too much. I'm not sure whether I told her about it but I rely on her to ring me up and tell me when it is. Unfortunately I think our wires got crossed so I missed it, and that was all my own fault though, no one else's. I didn't mean to because I have been trying really hard to go to all the appointments.
> *(21 year old male)*

> Well to be honest with you I have started missing a lot more now than before. The only reason why is that I just tend to forget because I have got so much on.
> *(19 year old male)*

Two respondents admitted that they would not intentionally fail to attend but had occasionally forgotten.

> I think I've missed like one appointment by accident, but I've never booked one and then just not bothered turning up.
> *(18 year old male)*

> I have missed some, I missed one when I got back from
> holiday but that was just because I totally forgot.
> *(18 year old female)*

Screening procedures

The procedures carried out at clinic appointments may make young people feel
they are under surveillance and, if they know their glycaemic control has been
poor, may put them off attending. Members of staff who were interviewed
described how sometimes it is difficult to communicate with young people at
clinic appointments. The hospital location, being busy, and the lack of privacy
all militate against a comfortable, relaxed consultation. Teenagers who do not
communicate can also make consultations awkward.

> It's very hard when people aren't speaking ... you're very
> conscious that you should be listening more than talking,
> but that's very hard if they won't talk back.
> *(Paediatric dietician)*

Persuading young people to discuss and modify their behaviour without
frightening them away from attending future appointments can be a difficult
balance to achieve. For young people, being told to take exercise, eat well and
test their blood regularly can be a 'hassle'.

> At one stage I was very overweight and every time I went to
> an appointment I was nagged at about my weight. My self-
> esteem plummeted. I stopped attending because I could not
> face them moaning about me putting on another pound.
> *(17 year old female)*

Young people are asked to test their blood sugar levels regularly at home and
record them in a booklet or on a computerised graph and to bring the results
to the clinic to discuss with staff. Diabetes specialist nurses are aware that some
young people are unwilling to do regular blood tests at home and may even
fabricate test results in order to fool staff and avoid being criticised.

> They hate blood tests. It's a reminder the whole time. It's to do
> with routine and they don't like anything to do with routine.
> *(Paediatric diabetes specialist nurse)*

At the large majority of clinic appointments, patients' HbA1c is measured, giving an average blood glucose level over a period of around three months. Some young people are nervous about the test and feel judged by staff if it is higher than the recommended level. In some cases they are afraid of being 'told off' so lie about blood tests carried out at home between clinic appointments. This feeling of being nagged, or even bullied, can be intimidating for some young people.

> I don't like the HbA1c tests because I worry that my blood sugar may be higher than they would like it to be.
> *(18 year old female)*

> I sometimes feel a little bit intimidated especially if my sugar control hasn't been brilliant.
> *(17 year old female)*

One young man was prepared to be told off:

> If my results are bad I sometimes think I am going to get a roasting if I go in so is it actually worth going in but I always think well, yeah, why not? If I know I have done something wrong it is never as bad as expected.
> *(20 year old male)*

Routine screening includes being weighed and measured and having injection sites checked. Patients are also asked to produce a urine sample for testing. Some young people feel self-conscious about being weighed, particularly if there is a lack of privacy. Many fail to bring in a urine sample or say they are unable to give one because they are embarrassed by the procedure. One young woman who logged onto the Diabetes Explained website described how teenagers may find personal questions uncomfortable.

> Teenagers are generally insecure about themselves and like to keep things to themselves. This can be impossible at clinic when you are asked every time – 'do you have your period? Is it regular? Do you smoke/drink? Are you sexually active? Are you following your diet properly?'… It's very off-putting to come to clinic and have to tell these things that their friends without diabetes can keep to themselves.

Team members also expressed awareness of how screening can be disagreeable for young people and of how ensuring that monitoring is carried out has to be done sensitively in order to maintain a rapport with the young person and not put them off attending next time.

> I mean getting your weight done, and your height done, and
> people talking about your details, that's fairly personal, and
> you can understand why people don't like that, and it is
> easier to pretend it's not there if you don't go to clinic, and
> don't do your blood sugars and so on.
> *(Paediatric dietician)*

Staff tread a fine line between supporting young people to monitor and
improve their glycaemic control and damaging their relationship with them.
Some were explicit that maintaining contact was sometimes more important
than good control. Without the contact, staff are unable to give young people
any help or advice at all.

> I think the bottom line is getting them to come to clinic.
> I mean, to me it doesn't matter what their control is like,
> you'll not get anywhere if you just don't get them to come,
> so the number one thing is getting them actually to attend.
> *(Paediatric dietician)*

'I don't see the point'

Some young people feel that there is little value in attending clinic
appointments because they say they are confident that they are able to look
after themselves without input from clinic staff. They may have been living with
diabetes for many years and believe that they have little more to learn. Younger
adolescents may be unwilling or unable to communicate with staff, while older
teenagers may feel they are too busy to attend and that coming to clinic
interferes with their notion of independence.

> I don't like going because I don't see the point as I know
> how to look after myself and it's really boring.
> *(15 year old female)*

> I don't really achieve anything at them, I don't think.
> I'd rather not have to go personally. I think they're
> pretty pointless.
> *(17 year old male)*

Others may prefer not to think about diabetes at all. The one persistent non-
attender in the sample confirmed this view.

> When I went to university, I think I went a bit in denial
> because I wanted to live my life how I wanted to and not
> have worries.
> *(22 year old male)*

Another university student, however, did 'see the point' but was not prepared to prioritise clinic appointments over other aspects of his life. Although he felt that staff at the new clinic he was registered with could give him good advice, he admitted that:

> I've been really slack actually. I mean my mum does tell me a
> couple of weeks before, and I tend to forget on the day or
> remember after it's happened or I have things to do on that
> day, so it's quite difficult to fit in. It's always been like there's
> been a rugby match on the night before and I'm too drunk
> to wake up in the morning or something stupid like that.
> When I did go the doctor said that he could devise this new
> programme for me which sounded really cool so I'd like to
> go and have a go at that and everything.
> *(20 year old male)*

Staff also recognised that some young people were unwilling to engage with diabetes but that this might be temporary and age related.

> For some it will be complete denial that they have something
> that needs attention so it will be a mixture of denial and
> they feel there is nothing to gain. Very often they then
> reappear sort of old and slightly more mature and it is often
> life events like girlfriends and getting engaged and getting
> married and stuff like that.
> *(Diabetes specialist nurse – adult service)*

A number of members of diabetes teams described how young people reappeared at clinic, having failed to attend for a couple of years. Greater maturity, fears about possible complications and life events, including pregnancy, were factors in patients deciding to make use of health services.

Views on non-attendance

When young participants in the study were interviewed for the second time, they were asked why they thought some people failed to attend clinic appointments. Some of them were regular attenders who valued clinic appointments, while others attended irregularly and sometimes reluctantly. They thought there were a number of reasons why people might fail to turn up.

Some thought young adults would feel they already knew enough about diabetes to need the reassurance or advice of professionals.

> I guess that they could feel that they're old enough now to deal with it themselves perhaps and they feel they don't need supervision as such.
> *(18 year old female)*

> They think so long as they've had it from a young age, they know what they are doing I suppose.
> *(18 year old female)*

> I think they think well, why should I sit there and get told what I already know.
> *(21 year old female)*

> I think it's because they don't like going. They don't see the point or they feel they don't need to.
> *(13 year old female)*

Others thought non-attenders might be too busy to go to the clinic, particularly if the waiting times were long.

> Maybe they are too busy. Obviously you have got a lot of responsibilities when you are older and things crop up at the last minute so sometimes you can't make it.
> *(18 year old male)*

Long periods between appointments meant people might forget to go.

> Maybe because the appointments are further apart, they tend to forget.
> *(15 year old female)*

Three felt that going to the clinic might be an intimidating or unpleasant experience.

Maybe they think that their control is not as good as it should be and they're worried that if they go to an adult clinic they won't get like the soft treatment.
(17 year old female)

Some people might just be in denial and don't want to acknowledge that something's wrong and they just want to tell you that it's not happening. Because I've known a few people who are diabetic and they've gone off the rails now and then, and then I think there are other people who are scared because they're going to say 'You can't eat this and you can't eat that, and you must stop smoking', you know, so I think there's that.
(20 year old female)

I suppose sometimes it can be a hassle getting there and sitting through a lecture. Sometimes it can feel that way and you are being told the best way to live your life and you think, 'OK but I don't want to'.
(21 year old male)

One suggested that going to an adult clinic where there was no one else of your age might be off-putting.

I think possibly from my own experience which is whenever I go in there I usually see people in the clinic and I don't think I have ever seen anyone else in my age bracket in there. It is all the sort of fifty plus and nothing to relate to there.
(23 year old male)

Another thought that moving to an adult clinic where one did not know the staff might make going to the clinic unattractive.

I think it's probably because they're used to being with certain people and having certain doctors and nurses and then having to change.
(17 year old female)

More than one said that it was up to individuals to choose whether or not to attend appointments and that non-attendance might not be a result of a particular clinic's structure or atmosphere.

> It's not necessarily something that the hospital does. I think
> it's probably an individual choice.
> *(19 year old female)*

The importance of family support

Young people were fulsome in their appreciation of the support received from parents and other family members. Although they sometimes considered their parents over-protective, they understood why parents were particularly concerned about their well-being. Apart from offering emotional and moral support, parents help young people by being well informed about diabetes, making sure family meals are suitable, collecting insulin supplies and accompanying their children to the clinic. The majority of young people (69 per cent) in the sample reported that a family member, in most cases their mother, took responsibility for ensuring that appointments with the clinic were made and kept. A third went to the clinic alone, while two-thirds went with a parent or, in one case, an older brother. Many of those who are accompanied by parents were given a lift to the hospital. Those who had moved to adult care were more likely than those using paediatric or adolescent services to go to the clinic alone but the difference was not large (45 per cent compared to 55 per cent).

It seems that parental support in terms of helping children and young people to deal with the day to day issues of living with diabetes and offering practical assistance to ensure that they maintain good glycaemic control is an important factor in young people keeping well. One young man described how his family's support has helped him deal with the condition.

> My family has been very supportive. I have read about some
> diabetics really hating it and I have never really hated myself
> having diabetes so I have just got on with it. I think that is partly
> because my parents have been so supportive … With hindsight,
> maybe, yes, they were over-protective but I can see why they
> were keen to get my control good and it was a good thing.
> *(20 year old male)*

Diabetes team members were also aware of the importance of family support for maintaining good control which includes attending clinic appointments. If young people are cared for and valued at home, they are more likely to look after themselves.

> I think a lot of the ones that don't come, it's to do with
> whether your parents are going to make you come or

remember. So it's a very dishevelled, scatty family where the children are left to look after themselves then they don't get supported in coming and because in that situation the child's left to their own devices and they're not looking after their diabetes.

(Paediatric diabetes specialist nurse)

Similarly a paediatrician, who cares for young people aged up to 15, identified family circumstances as key to clinic attendance and good control.

The majority of patients who have poor control I would say come from families which are disrupted or disorganised. And so if you have a patient who has a problem with attending regularly, or generally has poor overall control, it often reflects the family situation. And most of our patients, despite their age, are not responsible enough to decide to attend clinic on their own. They're always seen with the parent and if that parent doesn't see clinic as a priority, then nor will the child generally.

(Paediatrician)

Parents who have diabetes themselves may not feel it necessary for their child to attend clinic appointments. One nurse described how she encouraged a teenager to come to the clinic but that his mother, who also has diabetes, did not feel it was necessary because 'I know what I'm doing'. This presented a dilemma to the nurse who felt the young person was not being given a choice about whether or not to attend the clinic but was unable to discuss the issue with him as his mother was not in favour.

Administrative and organisational reasons for non-attendance

There may be administrative or organisational reasons why some young people fail to attend clinic appointments, particularly at the time of transition from paediatric to adult care. In some cases, young people may have to move from one hospital to another and the new hospital may be further from home. Adult clinics are less likely than adolescent services to be run in the early evening and it may be difficult for a young person to take time off from education or work, particularly at exam times. One young person said:

> That [missed appointment] was for college reasons. I think
> I've had to miss two because basically I had assessed
> practicals which obviously I certainly can't skive.
> *(21 year old male)*

> I had to miss an appointment early in the summer for an
> exam and then again at the beginning of the school year
> because it was my induction at university.
> *(18 year old female)*

One nurse told of a young man who had taken up a scarce apprenticeship after leaving school. He was concerned that taking time off from work to attend appointments might put him in a bad light with his employers particularly as he felt lucky to have been chosen for the training.

If procedures for transfer are not made clear, young people may be confused about where and when their first appointment is or may feel some trepidation about attending a new clinic, particularly if they do not know the staff. One respondent explained how she had missed an appointment when she moved to the adolescent clinic.

> It was at the time I was swapping round from the children's
> to the teenage clinic, and I was a bit unsure of what was
> going to happen.
> *(16 year old female)*

If they fail to turn up to more than one appointment, they may find they have been dropped from the register and will have to be re-referred by their general practitioner. Some clinic staff do their best to ensure this does not automatically happen.

> We are flexible about it. If there are some people that you
> know are having a difficult time, we will maybe say, 'Oh no,
> just keep sending that person an appointment' but say it is a
> 26 year old that's defaulted twice we will just send a letter to
> say another clinic appointment will not be sent unless your
> GP re-refers you. I think that happens on the third default
> appointment but for young people we kind of extend it a
> bit more.
> *(Diabetes specialist nurse – adult service)*

One nurse described how she tries to ensure that young people who attend the young adult clinic are not 'lost' even though, in some cases, it is difficult to ensure that they continue to use the service. Staff recognise that teenagers and young adults do not always behave responsibly in regard to their diabetes care and try their best to prevent them from slipping through the net.

> If they fail to turn up, I ring them basically. They will be sent another appointment. One of the advantages of being in this clinic is that they aren't treated like adults in that respect. If an adult patient fails to turn up on two occasions without cancelling the appointment a letter will go to the GP saying we're not sending for them anymore, refer back if you wish them to be seen and I think a letter goes to the patient as well to say that. In this clinic, they don't get discharged or I try and make damn sure they don't. That's why I don't like them getting out into the adult clinic before they should because if we're not on the ball and we've lost contact with them or if I'm assuming that somebody else is keeping tabs on them it doesn't always happen. They may slip through so it's not foolproof but in this clinic we will follow them up more rigorously. I will phone up or write to them or rebook them for the next clinic and then, if they then don't turn up, then I'll definitely be on their tail. Having said that some people are quite slippery. You can ring them any number of times and try and arrange to see them but if they don't want to see you then they won't.
> *(Diabetes specialist nurse – paediatric and adult services)*

Sometimes administrative systems break down and a few young people reported problems with being given an appointment. This is most likely to happen at transfer or when the young person has moved away to university and is more difficult to contact. One reported having problems of this nature:

> I've only been to one adult clinic and that was after I pestered them for an appointment … The appointment they gave me, the first one, I couldn't make so everything they gave me I said, 'no, I can't do that particular day or time' and then they just didn't send me one … I've kept on to them.
> *(18 year old female)*

Another described how she found it difficult to attend her first appointment in the adult clinic.

> My original appointment was 3 p.m. and then they changed
> it to half past five. I said, 'I can't make that. I go to work.' So
> she said, 'I can make you another one, or you'll just have to
> turn up and wait.' Well, I can't turn up and wait because I've
> got to get to work. I said, 'When will the next one be?' and
> she said, 'March.' I said, 'I think he's gonna want to see me
> before March.' I asked her why it was changed and she said,
> 'Well, you're an adolescent – adults take priority over you.'
> That was the receptionist's attitude.
> *(17 year old female)*

One young woman blamed the 'system' for difficulties at transfer to adult care.

> I think I just had problems with the transfer, changing over.
> Things didn't run smoothly like they're expected to and
> appointments were made wrong and things like that.
> I mean, you know, everybody makes mistakes.
> *(20 year old female)*

How clinic staff encourage young people to attend

Non-attendance at outpatient clinics is not confined to young people or to people with diabetes. Appointment dates are often sent months in advance which increases the likelihood of patients forgetting to attend. One study of four adult diabetes clinics in Australia found that if patients were sent a detailed information pack about their care before the appointment and were contacted by phone a week before, the non-attendance rate dropped dramatically, from 15 per cent to 1.4 per cent (Hardy *et al.* 2002). Another study of clinic bookings for adolescents also found that a telephone call on the eve of the appointment improved attendance rates. In this study default rates fell from 20 per cent to 8 per cent. 'Forgetting' was the most common reason given by patients who did not attend (Sawyer *et al.* 2002).

Clinic staff, particularly diabetes specialist nurses, who were interviewed were keen to maintain some contact with defaulters and, in some cases, tried a number of tactics to ensure that they continued to communicate with these young people. However, some health care staff felt that there was only so much they could do to attract people to clinic and recognised that, in the end, attending is a matter of personal choice. In the case of younger children, paediatric staff are prepared to follow child protection procedures if they are unable to maintain contact.

> We have a statutory obligation to see children with diabetes
> and we will go to court if necessary.
> *(Consultant paediatrician)*

Concerns about health risks faced by young people with diabetes have triggered a response from health care staff who want to ensure that clinics are acceptable to young patients and that they will turn up to appointments. Clinic structure, times and location, waiting times and the way patients are treated have all been considered by staff providing services for young people. Some nurses offer a flexible service for those who are unwilling to come to clinics.

> I've worked with teenagers who hate coming into clinic so
> the majority of times I will go out to them where they're far
> happier and it's a bit of I suppose bargaining goes on. Yes,
> I'm willing to make allowances and tailor the service to you
> but at the end of the day there's going to be occasions where
> you have to meet me halfway and come in. I tend to work in
> a manner where I'm chasing the whole time.
> *(Paediatric diabetes specialist nurse)*

Another described how she would approach a young person who had persistently failed to attend clinic appointments.

> We're not here to say, 'come back to the clinic, you need to
> see a doctor and have your bloods done'. I think we have to
> go in with the attitude that, 'well, it's your body, what do you
> want? How can we help?'
> *(Diabetes specialist nurse – paediatric and adult service)*

Despite the concern about young people's clinic attendance, staff admitted that there is no easy way of reducing the default rate. In one of the research areas, the team was exploring the possibility of employing a diabetes specialist nurse who would have responsibility for young people at the point that they made the transition to adult care. However, there was some scepticism about being able to provide a service that was attractive to all users. If a young person has made it clear that they are unwilling to attend hospital appointments, staff may suggest alternative services to ensure that they are receiving care.

> We will say, you know, we feel it's important that you have
> some contact with medical services and, if you don't want to
> come to our clinic maybe you should go and see your own
> doctor and arrange something else, that there are other
> clinics which you could go to, there are the satellite clinics,
> for example … I would be wanting them to have regular care
> and I'm not too bothered about where that care takes place
> so I want them to be within the service. If it's my clinic, that's
> fine, if it's a satellite clinic, well that's probably fine as well.
> *(Consultant paediatrician)*

Although patients of all ages may be taken off the clinic register if they fail to
turn up to two (or in some hospitals three) clinics, members of staff are
prepared to bend the rules in order to ensure young people remain within the
health care system. It is debatable at what age young people should be
considered as responsible adults and individual circumstances – developmental,
emotional, social and geographical – may be taken into account. One nurse
described how she worked hard to 'hang on' to unwilling patients.

> I make allowances as much as possible and go with the flow
> with them as opposed to saying 'you haven't attended clinic
> twice so you're off our books' sort of thing. I have worked
> with that system in my last hospital and hated it and I used
> to work the system and bring the kids back in by the back
> door so to speak.
> *(Paediatric diabetes specialist nurse)*

However, it may not be possible to continue to book people into oversubscribed
clinics when they continually default. One consultant felt that responsibility lies
with the patient to inform health care staff of their circumstances.

> Well, the norm in the adult clinic is if they fail to attend
> twice then they do get discharged because people don't tell
> us if they've moved away or if they've gone on prolonged
> holidays or gone somewhere for six months or gone away to
> university so, if they don't tell us, we don't know and we
> haven't got the facility to keep giving appointments to
> people who aren't going to use them. If people don't want
> our service but don't want to tell us they don't want it, we

can't accommodate them so we have to send them back to
their GPs or inform their GP and not reappoint them unless
we're asked to.

(Consultant diabetologist – adult service)

Our data, and evidence from the literature, show that some young people fail to
attend clinic appointments for a period of time but that the majority attend
regularly although many are likely to occasionally miss an appointment. Clinic
structure, a flexible approach, family support and health care staff maintaining
good relationships with young people are all factors in encouraging them to
attend but most young people will sometimes fail to turn up because they are
busy, ill or simply forget about the appointment. If it is clear that a young
person is unwilling to attend clinic appointments, staff may be prepared to offer
home visits or suggest alternative care. Carson and Kelnar (2000) argue that it is
important to maintain some form of contact with these young people 'however
minimal'. However, as noted above, it was not possible in this project to sample
a group of young people who persistently default from clinic attendance. We are
therefore unable to clarify why this minority of young people are unwilling to
keep in touch with diabetes services.

6. Transition to adult care

Guidelines for the optimal care of young people with diabetes stress the potential difficulties for adolescents of managing the progression to adulthood while living with a chronic illness and make recommendations for services tailored to meet the special needs of this age group. These guidelines suggest that transition from paediatric to adult care should be organised in such a way that young people are consulted before transfer and understand the process and implications of moving up to adult care.

The Consensus Guidelines produced by ISPAD (2000), for example, recommend that organised transfer to adult care should involve:

- negotiation and liaison between the paediatric and adult services including, when possible, the organisation of joint clinics;
- deciding on the optimal age and stage of development for transition to joint care or transfer to adult care depending on local services and agreements;
- preparing the adolescent for transfer in advance;
- ensuring that there is no hiatus in care at the time of transfer.

The principles of good practice for the care of young people with diabetes (British Diabetic Association 1995) stresses the importance of regular communication between paediatric and adult teams in ensuring that young people do not fall through the net of services. It also suggests that adult clinics could be age banded so that young people are able to attend with their peers. Results from a survey of paediatricians caring for young people with diabetes (Jefferson *et al.* 2003) found that respondents saw 45 per cent of 16 to 20 year olds in an age banded clinic and just over half (52 per cent) refer young people on to a young adult clinic.

It is widely acknowledged, therefore, that transition to adult care occurs at a time that can be difficult for young people with diabetes and that there is an increased likelihood that they might fail to regularly attend clinic appointments at the time of transfer and in the following months or years. Although there are no standardised procedures for managing the process of transfer, many hospital services have systems in place to ensure the best possible arrangements, depending on local resources and circumstances. There were, for example, jointly run clinics for young people in three of the hospitals included in the study.

The services described in this study have different arrangements for transferring young people from paediatric to adult care. All of them offer age banded clinics but the age at which young people become the responsibility of adult services and the availability of specialised transition services are variable. It is difficult in a qualitative study like this to identify which components of any particular service work best and therefore it is not possible to make firm recommendations for an ideal service. Young people who participated in the project had only experienced one kind of transition and so were not in a position to make comparisons. Unless individual young people had experienced particular problems with their diabetes care, they tended to accept the clinic arrangements and the move to adult care without reflecting on how the process could have been different. Some said that they missed staff from the paediatric clinic or that the move had been abrupt but they were able to accept the change in part at least because they had been offered no alternative. Most young people did not see clinic appointments as central to their lives and some regarded them as a necessary evil. Family life, friendships, social activities, education and employment were all more important to them than their more limited interaction with clinic staff.

However, this study has been able to highlight particular aspects of diabetes services and of transition to adult care that are critical to the quality of young people's experience at this important point in their lives. As noted above, almost all participants in the study were regular attenders at diabetes clinics and were, on the whole, positive about their experience of diabetes care. The study cannot claim to speak for those young people who do not attend clinics or who have no contact with diabetes services.

One cohort of young people was interviewed in the year before they moved to adult care and another in the year immediately after transfer. The majority was then interviewed again approximately a year later. Although most of those who were not yet in adult care at first interview had subsequently had at least one appointment with the adult service at the time of the second interview, some were waiting for their first appointment, and so effectively were between services, or were continuing to attend a jointly run adolescent or young adult clinic.

Preparation for transfer

The components of an effective transition programme as suggested by Russell Viner (1999) include a period of preparation when the young person is taught the necessary skills to manage their condition largely independently of adults. This would include the ability to manage their own treatment. The aim of this programme of education would be to ensure that young people are ready to attend an adult clinic where the ethos of care may be different from that which they have experienced in paediatric care. In the period leading up to transfer to adult care, Viner suggests that young people are introduced to the idea of moving on and that written material about the transition programme and the adult service should be made available.

The 42 young people included in the study who were attending an adolescent or transition clinic at first interview were asked what they knew about the adult clinic to which they would be transferring. As Table 6.1 shows, the majority did not know when or where the adult clinic was held or how often their appointments would be. A larger percentage knew where the adult clinic was held which is probably because it was in the same hospital as the one they were already attending or that they had been informed where it was held. None of the diabetes services included in the study produced a leaflet or any other literature about the transition process for patients although they did make available contact details for diabetes specialist nurses. Although clinic staff did not mention a systematic programme of education in self-management to prepare young people for transfer to adult care, staff interviewed in all services tailored care to meet the needs of young people although some admitted that they would benefit from both more resources and more expertise in terms of psychological support.

Table 6.1 Knowledge of adult clinic

Do you know...	when the adult clinic is held?		where the adult clinic is held?		how often appointments will be?	
	n	%	n	%	n	%
Definitely	6	14	11	26	1	2
Have some idea	3	7	7	17	6	14
Don't know	33	79	24	57	35	84
Total	42	100	42	100	42	100

The large majority were also ignorant of which doctor or nurse they would be seeing in the adult clinic (Table 6.2). None knew definitely which nurse they would see. More than half (55 per cent) said they had never met either the doctor or nurse they would be seeing (Table 6.3). Those who were attending a jointly run adolescent clinic should have met the adult consultant who would continue to see them in the adult clinic but this may not have been made clear to them.

Table 6.2 Do you know which doctor and nurse you will see at the adult clinic?

Do you know...	which doctor you will see?		which nurse you will see?	
	n	%	n	%
Definitely	3	7		
Have some idea	6	14	2	5
Don't know	33	79	40	95
Total	42	100	42	100

Table 6.3 Have you met the doctors and nurses at the adult clinic?

Have you met...	any of the doctors at the adult clinic?		any of the nurses at the adult clinic?	
	n	%	n	%
Yes, more than once	8	19	4	9.5
Yes, once	3	7	4	9.5
No	23	55	23	55
Not sure	8	19	11	26
Total	42	100	42	100

The replies to these questions show that most young people were not well prepared for transfer although two admitted that they might have been given information and forgotten it. It may be difficult for staff to gauge the optimal length of time for the period of preparation for transfer recommended by Viner as it may not be best practice to warn young patients that they will have to move to adult care while they still have two or more appointments in the adolescent clinic, particularly as appointments are three or four months apart.

All of the young people interviewed had some idea about the process of transfer to adult care but the extent and range of their knowledge varied widely. In some cases lack of information might mean that a staff member did not want to alarm a young person who might be nervous about moving; in others it might just be an oversight. In some areas, such as research area B, a cohort of young people moved up to adult care together as a group, but in others individuals might move because the timing of the adult clinic was more convenient for them or because caseload size meant there was pressure from younger patients joining the adolescent clinic from below.

Some young people described how the change had been explained to them by staff. The amount of information they were given and the point at which it was given varied.

> They said that I'd be changing over in the near future but they haven't really said much about it.
> *(16 year old female)*

> They did tell me I had two more appointments and then I would be moving up.
> *(17 year old male)*

> Basically they said it was the same as the teenage one but you were with more older people. About a year before they were saying, 'Oh, we're going to move you up to the adult clinic in about a year's time'.
> *(18 year old male)*

> Yeah, she spoke to me about it and she said, 'Do you mind? How do you feel about it? Would you rather stay here?' and she asked me whether it bothered me or not or whether I minded.
> *(17 year old female)*

> They said, 'You'll be going to the adult clinic. It'll be the next floor up, same doctor. No problem. We'll send your appointment through the post.' That was it. They didn't tell me what was going to happen and I just turned up expecting it to be the same. I think they might have given me a little leaflet or a bit of paper telling me something but they just said, 'You'll be going up to the adult clinic. I'll be your doctor. I'll see you there.'
> *(18 year old male)*

It would be helpful if the information young people are given about the transfer process was standardised so that all were given the opportunity to discuss it in advance and agree the timetable. Young people would like to know which members of staff they would see at the adult clinic, where and when the clinic is held and how often they were likely to be expected to attend. A leaflet with this information and contact numbers for staff could be given to them at their last appointment in the paediatric or transition clinic with, if necessary, a map of how to find the new clinic.

The transfer process

Russell Viner recommends that young people should be given detailed information about the programme of care offered by adult services and the opportunity to visit the adult clinic before their first appointment. Although a number of young people involved in the study had met doctors from the adult service at jointly run adolescent clinics, a formal visit to the adult clinic before transfer was not offered and nor did they receive detailed information about adult services. However, Viner's proposal that young people receive such detailed information about a year before transfer may not be the best suggestion. Young people admitted that they live in the present, sometimes forget their current consultant's name and may fail to take in information about their care arrangements. Even those in their twenties continue to make use of their mothers to remind them about appointments. It seems likely that information received a year before transfer may be lost or forgotten, or indeed be out of date, and that induction into adult care should happen shortly before transfer.

The 43 young people who were already attending an adult clinic at first interview were asked about how the transfer had been managed (Table 6.4). The majority said that they had not had the opportunity to discuss the transfer before moving up and did not have a choice about when to move. Nearly three-quarters said they had not met adult staff before transferring. Although just over half (53 per cent) said they had been told which doctor they would see when they moved up, nearly three-quarters said they did not know which nurse. The central role of specialist nurses in the care of young people with diabetes was stressed by many of those interviewed and it is likely that they would find it is as important to know which nurse they would see in adult care as which doctor.

Only a small minority (16 per cent) had had any choice about when to move. Although interviews with staff showed that in most hospitals there is some flexibility about when to refer young people to adult care, this has less to do with individual choice than with personal circumstances and health status. Clearly young people cannot remain in the care of paediatric departments indefinitely, especially as the pressure of numbers increases the paediatric caseload, but it should be possible for staff to discuss the timing of transfer with their patients early and to reassure them that they will continue to be cared for in an adult clinic.

Table 6.4 Preparation for transfer

	Yes		No		Total	
	n	%	n	%	n	%
Did you see a leaflet about the adult clinic?[1]	4	9	39	91	43	100
Had you met any of the staff beforehand?	11	26	32	74	43	100
Did you discuss the change beforehand?	15	35	28	65	43	100
Did you have a choice about when to move?	7	16	36	84	43	100
Did you know which doctor you would see?	23	53	20	47	43	100
Did you know which nurse you would see?	11	26	32	74	43	100

1 No research clinic produced a leaflet describing the transfer process although contact numbers for adult services were provided

Feelings about moving to adult care

Young people who attended an adult clinic when they were first interviewed were asked about how they felt about moving to adult care (Table 6.5). Despite the fact that more than half (58 per cent) did not feel they had been well prepared by staff and were not sure what to expect (51 per cent), the majority of these young people said they felt ready for the move and were not worried about it although only a minority (14 per cent) were pleased to be moving up. In almost all cases, these questions were asked after respondents had had experience of attending an adult clinic. This may have coloured their memory but it does seem that the majority of young people are resilient to change. Some may have missed well-known and well-liked members of staff from the paediatric department when they first made the move to adult care but this did not prevent them being willing to form new relationships with adult staff and making the best of the care they received.

Table 6.5 Feelings about moving to adult care

	Yes		No		Not sure		Total	
	n	%	n	%	n	%	n	%
Were you ready for the move?	36	84	6	14	1	2	43	100
Were you well prepared by staff?	17	40	25	58	1	2	43	100
Were you not sure what to expect?	22	51	20	47	1	2	43	100
Were you worried about the move?	4	10	38	88	1	2	43	100
Were you pleased to be moving?	6	14	34	79	3	7	43	100

Most seemed to accept the transition to adult care whatever their experience and did not see the move as a 'big deal'. This may be because they did not consider the clinic or clinic appointments to be a central feature of their lives.

> It doesn't really bother me, if you know what I mean, it is just a place where you have to go every once in a while.
> *(15 year old female)*

> I haven't really thought about it. I'm not really bothered about moving. It doesn't bother me.
> *(17 year old female)*

> I mean, people change doctors. It's no different to anything else that changes.
> *(20 year old female)*

However, some who had not yet transferred did have concerns about the move. They were either afraid that the adult clinic would be busier than the one that they were attending and that they would therefore have less time to consult with staff at appointments. Some were worried about losing contact with staff whom they liked and trusted.

> The old clinic was quite quiet. I imagine this one's going to be much more busier and packed I guess. Before it used to be just me there. It's not going to be like that.
> *(17 year old female)*

I'm not worried but I suppose more wondering about it. Going from the younger one to the older one. Is it going to be more busy? Are they going to worry about you more or less?
(17 year old male)

I'll have less time. There will be more people. I don't mind moving but I feel the adolescent clinic is better because they talk to you more. I like the level of conversation from the staff at the adolescents', not adult to adult kind of thing.
(16 year old male)

The concern about leaving well-known staff members was linked to worries about what the adult staff might be like.

I wouldn't want to move because I wouldn't know if [the nurse] would be there or not.
(16 year old female)

It's going to be different. New to me. I'm not really worried but a bit worried about what the staff are going to be like.
(17 year old male)

I prefer to leave it how it is but I know that it does have to change. It's that I've got used to the people from the clinic.
(17 year old female)

It will be a lot easier to get to but it's just having to get to know the doctors and having the confidence in them to tell them things and stuff.
(15 year old female)

One was pragmatic about losing contact with the paediatrician and acknowledged that getting to know a new doctor was a two-way process – you know them but they also know you!

I would be a bit less comfortable at first, I think, because I don't know [the adult doctor] that well and I just think that [the paediatrician] knows who I am and everything about me. I would get to know him in time I suppose. It's not a major problem.
(17 year old female)

Some young people who were attending appointments in the adult service felt they could have been better prepared by staff. They felt moving had been difficult, perhaps more difficult than they had expected. Leaving staff whom they may have known for many years was a factor for some, while others felt rejected by paediatric staff because they had not had the opportunity to discuss the move or influence its timing in any way.

> I think you should have a choice of when you want to move.
> They just told me that I would be going. I didn't have a choice.
> *(17 year old female)*

> I think it is a bit too much of a big jump from one to the other. It felt a bit too quick, the changeover.
> *(17 year old female)*

> They weren't that bad, they did tell me when I was going and stuff but they didn't really explain what the difference was. I think that's what they need to do. Explain the difference between the children's and the adults and then it wouldn't be quite such a shock when you go there. Because when you are actually there it's not that much of a difference really.
> *(18 year old female)*

> The nurses and everything are lovely now, but I think that stage of actually changing probably were the worst part of it.
> *(19 year old female)*

> I think I'd probably have preferred to stay [in the transition clinic] but I think that was only because I knew the people. I think it probably was the right time.
> *(17 year old female)*

However, having made the move to adult care, a number of young people were happy with the adult service particularly if they responded well to the extra responsibility they felt it brought.

> Since I have moved to the adult diabetic clinic, I have learned a bit more about diabetes and I feel I can talk to them better than I did at the children's hospital. I think I have been handling my diabetes better now that I am at the adult clinic.
> *(16 year old male)*

> I preferred going up to the adult clinic. Being with people
> more my age, the learning of new stuff and that and the
> clinic as a whole being about diabetes and not like a hospital
> all full of different sorts of things. No other things on their
> minds. They can talk to you, one to one about diabetes.
> *(18 year old male)*

Another, who had moved to adult care, felt that moving up had been part of a strategy to help him take more responsibility.

> I was a bit worried. Everything was on a plate for me in the
> children's one. They just gave me what I wanted. That was
> the idea – to move up to get a grip on myself. I was sorry to
> leave the children's but I was glad that they thought I was
> mature enough to go to the adults.
> *(17 year old male)*

Young people responded differently to being offered more responsibility. Although the majority preferred to be treated like an adult, some found it difficult to handle. One described how she did not feel ready for making decisions for herself.

> I was getting treated like a baby at [the children's hospital]
> and I preferred like being told what to do and not saying,
> 'what do you think you should do?'. At [the children's
> hospital] they were telling me what to do. Now they expect
> me to do stuff for myself.
> *(16 year old female)*

The fact that older people attended the adult clinic was commented on by some respondents. Although in principle they did not 'mind' sitting in a waiting room with people much older than themselves, some found it uncomfortable or depressing.

> There's not very many people at the clinic I go to now that
> are my age and it's depressing, the atmosphere,
> unfortunately, with what they're talking about.
> *(19 year old female)*

> It was more frightening because I was sat there looking at all
> these older people thinking, 'that's going to happen if I
> don't control it' and watching a lot of them struggling to
> walk. It was scary actually. But it told me what could happen.
> It livened me up.
> *(20 year old female)*

The ideal transition

Young people were asked to identify an ideal method of transfer to adult care from a list provided by the interviewer. The options were:

- an adolescent clinic for young people aged 13 to 18 years old where you see both the doctor from the children's clinic and the 'adult' doctor for at least a year;
- a clinic run by a specialist adolescent doctor for people aged between 13 to 18 years old;
- a young adult clinic staffed by an 'adult' doctor for people aged 18 to 25;
- one handover meeting between you, the children's doctor and the 'adult' doctor;
- a letter from the children's clinic to the adult clinic introducing you but with no joint meeting;
- the nurse from the children's clinic accompanies you to the first appointment at the adult clinic and introduces you to staff there.

None of those interviewed were in favour of the transfer process being simply a letter of referral from one doctor to another except as a formality or if it was not possible for a patient to attend a handover clinic. Young people were much more likely to value continuity of care and a staged transition in age banded clinics. It has not been possible to quantify responses as, in many cases, young people qualified their answers depending on what they saw as many possible circumstances. However, the large majority favoured an adolescent clinic where it would be possible to get to know staff from the adult service before finally saying goodbye to paediatric staff followed by a young adult clinic. One 18 year old female, however, was concerned that seeing two doctors either consecutively or together might be confusing.

> They [the doctors] will be discussing what's going on but they might tell you something different and it's going to leave you in the middle wondering what to do. I think it would be best if you just stick with the one doctor. Then they can concentrate more on you and you can concentrate more on them.

A 21 year old male, who was still attending an 'adolescent' clinic, preferred to continue to see the same doctor.

> I think it's good to stay with the same doctor for as long as
> possible. I don't think you should rush the transfer. I'd like
> to stay at this clinic a bit longer before they transfer me onto
> the adult one because if you build a relationship with one
> doctor, there's no point breaking that relationship and
> going to another one and going through all that shit again.
> Especially when one doctor knows all the stuff about you
> and how you cope and everything.

Although two respondents acknowledged that frequent changes in insulin dose
and the stress of exams make the teenage years a difficult period to cope with
diabetes and that therefore a specialist adolescent doctor might be helpful at
this time, few were in favour of this option because they thought it might entail
changing doctors more often than the traditional single move from paediatric
to adult services. It may also be that most respondents had not come across an
adolescent specialist and did not choose this option for that reason.

Age banded clinics were favoured by all although there was variation in
precisely when respondents thought transfer should happen. Most agreed that
attending an adolescent clinic from 13 to 18 was appropriate and then a young
adult clinic up to 25 years. Twelve respondents felt that there should be
flexibility about when the transfer should happen and that patients should be
consulted about when they felt ready to make the move.

> I think people should go when they are ready.
> *(17 year old female)*

> It should be the client's choice. I mean if you don't feel
> that you want to move up yet then you should be able to
> stay with them.
> *(17 year old female)*

> It depends. Every individual is different. I think we should
> be able to choose when we're meant to change over really,
> when we feel we're ready enough.
> *(16 year old female)*

> I guess around 17 or 18 is ideal. Perhaps you could have
> leeway at either end. Let people choose.
> *(18 year old female)*

Two young women used their own experience to illustrate this point. One thought that her attitude towards diabetes had been mature since childhood and that it therefore might have been appropriate for her to transfer to adult care before some of her peers.

> I think it's going to vary. I always liked to know a lot and, even when I was in the children's one, I liked to change my own insulin and things like. So I could have gone earlier, whereas some people, they still have difficulty.
> *(22 year old female)*

The other was a young mother and felt that her experience meant that she should be treated as an adult older than her years.

> I think it would be a good idea as long as they didn't generalise you, you know, just because you're that age put you in that clinic. I think really it's a better idea to judge people on their maturity, their situation, their life rather than their age because I'm treated like a 19 year old mother, not a 19 year old. I've probably gone through a lot more than most others.
> *(19 year old female)*

The expertise in dealing with young people by staff in adolescent units or clinics was acknowledged by young people, as was the difference in their approach compared to that of staff in children's clinics. They valued the fact that they are able to talk openly to staff about their lifestyles and expected to have more say in their care than they did when they were younger without being 'told off'.

> Up till you're about 13 or something you follow what your parents say, and you give injections religiously, you do it like that, but from then you think, 'Oh no, I'm not going to do it'. You sort of get rebellious or something, and then you stop and they don't know what to do and then if you're at a children's unit, they're sort of like, 'Well, you've done it before and you can do it again', that sort of thing, but if you go to the adolescent one, they go, 'We know, we understand it's hard' and stuff, so it's their speciality really in that age group. It helps.
> *(18 year old female)*

Young people also favoured being transferred to a young adult clinic when they moved to adult care. They acknowledged that growing up is a gradual process and that there is no magic point at which young people become adult and that therefore services should also be sensitive to this process. Attending a clinic with others of the same age group was also seen as being helpful because one could learn from others' experiences.

> I would say 20 rather than 18. I would say 19 is a bit too young to be thrown into the adult clinic. Not talking about 19 being an adult but 19 diabetes wise being treated amongst the adult diabetics.
> *(21 year old male)*

> Where you're not quite a kid, but you're not quite one of them cold adults that knows what they're doing and just comes in for a regular check up. So you do need something between that.
> *(20 year old male)*

> I think as long as you know there's people your own age kind of in similar situations. A young adult one would be quite handy because by the time I went there, there would have been other people there who had a wider perspective about it. Things that I haven't necessarily done, or wouldn't be doing myself, but you'll still kind of get help from that experience.
> *(18 year old female)*

Viner (1999) suggests that disease based programmes serve patients best and that 'transition programmes are poorest where no specific adult services exist'. However, he argues that transferring young people to general diabetes clinics is not a good idea because of the 'obese, elderly, sick patients populating these clinics' and therefore advocates the development of young adult clinics. One 22 year old male agreed, saying that he would prefer not to attend the same clinic as much older people who might be experiencing complications of diabetes.

> I don't mind up to say 40. But you don't really want to go there seeing loads of old people with awful problems. You don't want to see that really.

The interviews with young people included in the study show that they are in favour of a 'smooth transition of care from paediatric diabetes services to adult diabetes services', as described in Standard 6 of the National Framework for Diabetes (DH 2001). The essential elements of such a transition as identified by both the literature and young people are preparation before transfer, adequate information about the procedures at transfer, a measure of continuity of care, some flexibility about the timing of transfer, age banded clinics and a changing approach by staff as patients mature. Young people who attended the adolescent unit in research area E were appreciative of the fact that it catered for their age group, recognising the staff's special skills in working with young people. Clearly the availability of resources and caseload sizes will have an effect on how individual services are able to operationalise the Standard but there is evidence from the six services included in the study that the necessity of managing this transition effectively is recognised by health care professionals and that, in many places, efforts are being made to offer a 'smooth transition'.

7. Services for young people with diabetes – the professional perspective

As noted above, guidelines for the care of young people with diabetes make recommendations for the type and quality of care young people should receive from the health service and how the transition from paediatric to adult care should best be managed. It has already been suggested that there are a number of structural adjustments that can be made by diabetes teams to comply with these guidelines – such as the age banding of clinics for young people, for example – but the personal approach of members of staff is also key in creating a rapport with young people. Interviews with members of staff who work with young people in the six research areas identified a number of the issues that they considered central to forming positive relationships with young people. These included the importance of both staff and young people being honest, working in partnership both as a multidisciplinary team and with young people, involving parents and meeting information needs, including discussing complications of diabetes. This chapter focuses on the particular issues facing health care staff who work with young people with diabetes.

Treating adolescents is not the same as treating younger children or adults. The adolescent years can be difficult for all young people and living with a chronic illness can make the change from child to adult more stressful. The ability of teenagers to take responsibility for their own diabetes management will depend on their stage of development and their individual characteristics and circumstances. Some may feel ready to take on more self-care but not be organised or rigorous enough to do it in reality. Others, particularly those who are newly diagnosed, may be overwhelmed just coping with the day to day challenges of diabetes. Some may want more independence than their parents are willing to allow, causing possible family conflict and resulting in stress which can interfere with self-care and glycaemic control (Miller-Johnson *et al.* 1994). Of course, many young people with diabetes manage the transition to adulthood with few problems but it is recognised that glycaemic control can deteriorate during this period (see for example Bryden *et al.* 2001). Young people with diabetes are also more likely to become overweight in adolescence (Bryden *et al.* 1999) at a time when they are especially self-conscious about body image. The physiological changes they go through, combined with their increasingly independent lifestyles and the stresses of school work, mean that these young people are a distinct group with particular problems and needs.

The link between tight glycaemic control and the long-term health of people with type 1 diabetes was confirmed by the Diabetes Control and Complications Trial (1993). The monitoring of control is therefore a central function of consultations between health care staff and young people with diabetes with the aim of maintaining or improving blood glucose levels. Young people, however, may face difficulties in maintaining good control, or may be unable or unwilling to alter their lifestyles to make it possible. Their understanding of their own adherence to treatment may also be at odds with that of health care professionals (du Pasquier-Fediaevsky and Tubiana-Rufi 1999). Puberty is associated with increased insulin resistance which makes it especially challenging for adolescents to obtain good control. Health professionals should aim to help patients alter their behaviour in order to improve control while allowing them to enjoy the quality of life of a 'normal' teenager.

Staff should also be aware of the effect of living with diabetes on their patients' psychological health. There is evidence that adults with diabetes are more likely to suffer from depression than those in the general population (Lustman *et al.* 1992) and one study has shown that girls with diabetes are more likely to suffer from symptoms of anxiety and depression than are boys (La Greca *et al.* 1995a). Studies have shown that behavioural problems in adolescence seem to be important in influencing glycaemic control in young adulthood (Bryden *et al.* 2001). Psychosocial factors also play an integral role in the management of diabetes in both children and adults (Delamater *et al.* 2001). The psychological functioning of young people with diabetes is linked to glycaemic control and so it is important that this is taken into account by health care staff who should refer young patients to psychological services when appropriate.

How do members of diabetes teams balance the sometimes conflicting tasks of encouraging young people to improve control while allowing them to take an increasingly central role in their own care? Team members who were interviewed for this study described how they communicate with young people and the difficulties they sometimes face. Staff members acknowledged that, because diabetes is a chronic condition that must be treated daily, young people (and their parents) are central to ensuring their own well-being and so the management of their care must be a partnership between staff, parents and young people themselves. Health care staff tread a fine line between ensuring that young people are aware of the consequences of poor glycaemic control and not threatening them and, perhaps more dangerously, frightening them away from clinic appointments altogether.

One of the difficulties in treating young people is that relatively high blood glucose levels may not affect the way they feel in the short term and it may be hard therefore to persuade them of the seriousness of persistent poor control.

> We wouldn't have a problem if everybody felt bad as soon as their blood sugar went up. Actually they only feel bad, most of them, when their blood sugar is too low. Those who don't feel OK with high blood sugar actually have an advantage if you like because they will do something about it.
> *(Consultant diabetologist)*

The fact that young people with poor control may feel well, combined with their perception that they are indestructible, means that health care staff have to constantly find ways of encouraging them to look after themselves. Their approach encompasses education, talking about diet and lifestyle, adjusting treatment to suit individuals, ascertaining young people's own commitment to improved control, cajoling and, sometimes, threats.

Honesty – the best policy

As mentioned above, the aim of monitoring glycaemic control is to avoid the risk of long-term medical complications. In order to ensure that young patients understand the dangers, staff are prepared to talk to them about the risks of poor control while being careful not to frighten them. The team at hospital E, for example, have an explicit policy of being honest with their young patients in the hope that they will reciprocate and tell the truth about how they look after themselves between appointments. Staff would prefer young people to be honest even if they have failed to monitor their blood at home, have omitted insulin or are smokers. Young people should not feel the need to fabricate test results in order to avoid being 'told off' by staff.

> I mean of course my main aim is to get HbA1c's down and to prevent complications and so on but I don't think that will happen unless we do build up a relationship with people and they feel that there's trust there and honesty. I think the biggest tool you can have is honesty because they know when somebody's trying to patronise them and they don't like that, and I wouldn't like that either.
>
> *(Paediatric dietician)*

This policy can sometimes be difficult to put into practice.

> We have to always obviously be honest with the patients as we would hope they would be honest with us. Often they are not honest with us and we have to try and find a way to tell them that we know they're not being honest – it's often a bit of a game. But what we want is to be able to speak frankly with them about their condition, and I think the hardest thing is to make them realise that even if they ignore their diabetes now, they are making decisions now about the rest of their lives. It's not intended to be us versus them, it is supposed to be all the people in the room versus diabetes as opposed to having the patients feel that they have to jump through hoops for us.
>
> *(Paediatrician)*

One doctor talked about adolescents' understanding of risk and how it develops.

> It is clear that their ability to understand and conceptualise risk changes as also does their ability to understand that it applies to them. If you look at the development of adolescent thinking, their ability to understand risk develops but initially they can understand the risk but they don't believe it applies to them. That's the kind of bulletproof thinking that adolescents have. So we have to constantly come back to talking about complications.
>
> *(Consultant paediatrician)*

Sometimes staff feel it is necessary to be brutally honest with patients in order to make them understand the risks of poor control, though they are careful not to threaten but to look at ways to make improvements.

> We will sometimes be very hard on patients and the families,
> other times we will be very sympathetic, but we have a very
> strong policy of honesty and we don't head pat.
> *(Consultant paediatrician)*

To illustrate this, one paediatrician talked about a particular consultation he
had had with a teenager and his mother. The teenager's control had been poor
for some time and he told them that if it did not improve then there would be
serious consequences. He made it clear that he shared responsibility for
improving the situation and was careful not to be critical of the teenager or his
mother. Both left the hospital very upset and the doctor received a phone call
from the boy's father asking what had happened. He described how:

> I spoke with him quite straight and, two days ago, one of my
> colleagues received a phone call from the same father who
> said this was the best consultation that they'd ever had, that
> the adolescent and the family had been told some home
> truths, and that they were examining their whole approach
> to diabetes care... If you'd asked me ten days ago what did I
> think of that consultation, I would have told you it was a
> disaster. If you ask me today, I would tell you that it went
> really well. So I don't think we do anyone any favours if,
> when they come through the door, we pat them on the head
> and say, 'There, there, you're doing fine, off you go, we'll
> see you in four months'. I think that's a waste of time.

A nurse talked about a similar consultation and its result.

> I think most of the nurses don't put the fear of God or the
> fear of renal failure into them. I did have a phone call from
> a mother the other day who'd just seen one of the paediatric
> registrars for an older child coming to the paediatric clinic.
> It was a teenager of 13 or 14 and the registrar had said, 'If
> you carry on like this you're going to end up in a wheelchair
> or with no kidneys' or whatever. That filled me with horror
> to begin with but the mother said it's maybe what the boy
> needed and then we went in there with the softly approach
> and the nurse did a home visit. So put the fear in and then
> put the support in.
> *(Diabetes specialist nurse – paediatric and adult services)*

There are advantages for young people when they feel they can be honest with staff. If they are prepared to admit to their level of commitment to regular blood testing, for example, staff can then help them match their treatment to their ability and willingness to undertake tests. Changing the number of daily insulin injections and/or the type of insulin used, for example, can allow the young person more flexibility and spontaneity while improving their glycaemic control.

> I try and encourage people to think that diabetes shouldn't control them, but you can't take it away so you have to respect it. You have to try and find a balance where you can keep it under control but still have your independence and the lifestyle that you choose to lead. You can try and minimise the damage. If they can be honest with us and tell us what they want to do then we can maybe help them solve some of the problems. For example, if they didn't want to eat breakfast or if they wanted to go out clubbing. If they're honest with us then we can surely try and work around these problems.
> *(Diabetes specialist nurse – adult service)*

Working in partnership with young people

Staff who were interviewed explained how they try to ensure that young people understand how to look after themselves and consult them about the best treatment regimen for them as individuals. Diabetes care includes a combination of education, support, dietary advice and the adjustment of insulin types and doses to allow young people to live more flexibly and spontaneously. Staff offer new devices such as insulin pens and up-to-date blood testing meters as they become available, ensuring that patients are taught how to use them. A successful regimen is one that allows the young person to achieve good control and to live without unreasonable restrictions. This is likely to be more effective than a rigid one which the young person finds too onerous and so does not stick to.

Staff were clear that there was little point in imposing unrealistic goals on young people but attempted to work together with them to encourage health enhancing behaviours. This means that staff have to know enough about the young person's lifestyle and capabilities to help them fit treatment around what is feasible for the individual.

We don't tell people what to do, we ask them what is reasonable for them, what is a realistic goal for them to achieve. How often they need to do blood sugars, for example. I will personally ask them what is realistic for them and, if they say one a week, I will accept that.
(Diabetes specialist nurse – adult service)

I want to find out what they expect. I want to find out if they think anything has to change. I want to know what they are going to do to facilitate change because sometimes people say, 'Well, what are you going to do about that?' And really the answer is, 'Well, what are you going to do about it?' Because I can do a bit but I can't do it all.
(Diabetes specialist nurse – adult service)

We very much try and put the onus onto them. There's no point in us being paternalistic about it. It would be very easy for us to say 'Look, phone us up once a week, we will have a look at your blood sugars, we will make changes to your insulin dose'. That would be very easy and they may come to clinic and have the best control in the world but their quality of life might be zero. So we try to get them to make the decisions.
(Paediatric diabetes specialist nurse)

I suppose the real emphasis of the clinic is to try and look at what the young people want, and what their goals are, and then try and motivate them to shift their goals. It's about matching goals. That's the ethos of the clinic.
(Consultant paediatrician)

It must be a joint decision. We can only advise I think and give them as much information as they're able to take on board, but they must make the decisions themselves as to what's right for them. I mean we obviously help them towards the right decisions and maybe try to get them on the right path, but it must be what they want to do or they won't do it anyway. And it's quite good to sort of problem solve with them to see what would suit them best. I mean there's all sorts of theory, but it's not always possible to put it into practice.
(Dietician – adult service)

It is important that the adolescent understands that the responsibility is shared between themselves, their family and the diabetes team. Staff say they want young people to seek their advice and make use of their expertise and recognise that the young person's feelings about diabetes and diabetes care may change depending on circumstances, mood and well-being.

> One of the things we now understand more about
> adolescents is that they don't like to be just dumped with all
> the responsibility, nor do they like to have none, and that
> feeling changes and so we need to be flexible.
> *(Consultant paediatrician)*

One of the difficulties for staff is that young people may feel that adults simply 'don't understand'. They may have different priorities, be embarrassed about talking to adults who they see as in authority and be unwilling to engage with members of staff.

When asked when she felt a consultation had been successful, one member of staff said:

> When you get the adolescent to talk to you. When you see
> them beaming and not hiding under their baseball caps. You
> can always tell their control's rotten if they've got a baseball
> cap on. I'm not joking! They come in scowling. And the
> parent and the child are sitting with their backs to each
> other. You know it's gone pretty well if you've got more than
> a grunt out of them.
> *(Paediatric dietician)*

Another described how she tries to understand what it is like to be young and how young people's lifestyles might make good glycaemic control difficult to achieve.

> I try and put in perspective the effects of poor control but at
> the same time I try and bear in mind that their viewpoint is
> entirely different from mine. The last thing you want to do is
> alienate yourself from the young person but at the same
> time I feel I do have a responsibility to make them aware
> that there are consequences of poor control but fully
> understand how difficult it is to be out all night at a party
> and be diabetic. So I try and be realistic about how difficult

it is especially if they have just moved to uni or just moved to
college or just started drinking. To say to a 16 year old boy
that you are not allowed to drink is just daft. So I do try and
be realistic but at the same time I don't lose sight of the fact
that we have a responsibility to try and motivate and achieve
good control.
(Diabetes specialist nurse – adult service)

The majority of young people interviewed for the study felt that doctors and
nurses understood their point of view. A few felt they did not.

I had someone else as a doctor before and he saw everything
from the way that somebody from his perspective would see
it. He didn't see all the problems that I would face being my
age, being diabetic and having to go to school. The doctor I
have now, he can understand that sometimes you might be
in a rush and you might not have time to take your blood
sugars in the morning or you just might not be bothered or
you might just not feel like doing it. He can understand how
somebody of my age would feel about having diabetes. I just
think he is a lot more understanding and I can connect a lot
more. It's almost as he is like a friend in the same position as
me. That's the way I see it.
(18 year old male)

The same young man also felt he had a good relationship with the diabetes
specialist nurse which meant he could be honest with her.

I will just say she is very open. She gives the impression you
can talk to her. The top one as well, you can have a laugh
with her so it doesn't feel so formal when you are speaking
to her like you would do a doctor. You don't feel like you
need to show you are really in good control, you can just like
say what you are doing to her.

A 16 year old girl who made contact with the research team through the
'Diabetes Explained' website had had a different experience.

I tend not to attend clinics. This is because I know what
I have to do to get my blood sugars at a reasonable level.
I found when I used to go, they didn't ask 'What can I do

to help?', they just said, 'Why aren't you doing it?' Diabetics
need to be encouraged, especially young teenagers, and our
consultants should be there to help, not tell you off every
time you go to see them.

Involving parents

Although the majority of young people attended clinic appointments with a
parent, over half consulted with the doctor (51 per cent) and nurse (57 per
cent) on their own. Staff were keen for young people to take increasing
responsibility for managing their condition but did not want to exclude parents
if the young person wanted them present. In order to allow young people
autonomy but not to banish parents from the consultation, most members of
staff encouraged, but did not pressurise, the young person to consult alone first
and then invited the parent into the room. One of the reasons for an individual
consultation is to allow young people to talk privately about sensitive issues,
such as smoking and drinking alcohol, without a parent present, which might
inhibit them from speaking openly.

> I actually do my best to see them on their own. I will let the
> parent in later if necessary. Because there are things that
> kids will tell you on your own that they will not tell you in
> front of a parent. I need to ask them if they drink, if you are
> 13 you are going to say 'No' if your mother is sitting beside
> you and it is really important to know that.
> *(Diabetes specialist nurse – adult service)*

> Obviously things like sex, smoking and alcohol are probably
> going to be no-go areas with a parent there, so I think the
> best compromise really is to have time with the parent and
> time without the parent in the same visit.
> *(Diabetes specialist nurse – adult service)*

Both parents and young people may feel more comfortable with this
arrangement when they have got to know staff at the clinic. This is particularly
true when young people first move to adult services.

> I don't have a set policy that I insist on seeing the patient on
> their own, although that is what I prefer to do. Very often

for the very first visit both the parent and the child come in
and then once I think they have both met me and they both
feel a bit more happy then I will work towards just seeing the
child on their own and seeing the parent afterwards.
(Diabetes specialist nurse – adult service)

One doctor preferred to invite the young person and their parent into the
consultation first and then talk alone to the young person.

As much as possible we try and encourage them to come in
alone and often I'll interview them together and separately
in the same situation so I might say to the parent, I might
just get them both in and say, 'How're we getting on?' and
then I might say to the parent, 'There are a few things I
want to discuss with Michael. Would you mind if we just
had a chat? There are a few growing up things I want to
talk to him about.' There are things like alcohol and
smoking and drugs.
(Consultant diabetologist – adult service)

While wanting to encourage their patients' independence and provide
confidentiality, staff were also conscious of the importance of family support for
young people with diabetes and did not want to alienate or offend parents.
Sometimes they found it difficult to interpret what the young person or the parent
would find most comfortable and tried to be flexible in order to accommodate
possibly conflicting needs. Sometimes a young person might discuss an issue that
the doctor or nurse felt the parent should know about. In these cases, staff would
seek the young person's permission before sharing it with a parent. However, staff
acknowledged how important parents are for their children's self-care and said
they would prefer parents to know if there were any problems.

I find that quite difficult to handle really I confess. I think that
the child, the young person, ought to be independent, ought
to be able to discuss with me confidentially and I think if I felt
that there was something that maybe parents should know
about I would ask the young person what they felt about that
and whether I ought to be discussing it with a parent. I don't
think it's happened very often really but mostly they are quite
willing that we tackle it with a parent and occasionally not. If
they're not happy I wouldn't discuss it.
(Consultant paediatrician)

> Sometimes the teenager wants to come in on their own and,
> if they want to, that's fine. In that case sometimes the parent
> will ring later and that's always a difficult one. I understand
> their concerns. I don't give out any confidences but would
> talk about the way we're going and things.
> *(Diabetes specialist nurse – paediatric and adult service)*

> We have an open, flexible approach. A lot of kids don't want
> their parents in with them and clearly what we are trying to
> do is to concentrate on the patient so I say, 'Mum and dad
> can come in if they want to' and, if they say, 'Oh no!', that is
> fine, they don't come in. If that does happen and I think
> there is a problem I might well go and say to the parents,
> 'Look, so-and-so is not doing quite so well but these are the
> things we are planning to do' so I make sure the parents are
> somehow involved with the managing. If the young person
> said to me, 'Don't talk to mum and dad', I wouldn't.
> *(Consultant diabetologist – adult service)*

Parents were more likely to be part of a consultation in paediatric clinics than in
transition or adult ones and young people seemed to welcome their presence
because they felt that parents were more likely to remember what questions to
ask and what had been said afterwards. One young woman explained how
useful it was to have her mother present.

> I did find that when I went with my mum, she used to ask a
> lot more questions about things, which brought up more
> issues as well. I would actually find out more, probably,
> because I don't really ask a lot now but maybe that's just
> because I know more. She used to have more concerns
> about, say, if we were going on holiday she would ask about
> ten thousand questions about what should we do, what
> should we take, that I wouldn't think to ask.
> *(18 year old female)*

Sometimes, however, staff felt that parents were taking too prominent a role and
would not allow the young person to speak for themselves.

> But sometimes it's not appropriate and sometimes parents
> insist on coming in and you can see that they're not wanted
> by their offspring and then it's difficult because you tend to

have a sullen person sitting there who might otherwise make
a bit more for themselves of the consultation. A lot of it
comes down to knowing the families I think.
(Diabetes specialist nurse – paediatric and adult service)

One nurse felt able to talk to a mother about giving her son more autonomy.

One of the parents … you could see that she was very
reluctant to let her power go if you like. The mother wanted
to answer the questions the whole time. The child was
perfectly capable but was obviously familiar with the scenario
in as much as he would look at his mum and then let his
mum do all the talking. He knew what he was talking about
and could quite easily cope without her there but she
wanted to do it. The mum herself recognised what she was
doing and then we talked a little bit about her letting go and
allowing the child to do all of the things that he wanted to
do without her involvement.
(Paediatric diabetes specialist nurse)

One young man described the advantages of seeing the doctor without his mother.

I know the doctor wanted me to go there without my mum.
It made a difference because they could talk to me. Before
they would ask me a question and my mum would answer it
before I could say anything. So, yeah, I suppose it did make
a difference. It made it more of a one to one where I could
get something across and they could get something across.
Before they would get something across and my mum would
get there before I could get anything back.
(19 year old male)

The question of whether parents should be present at consultations can be a
sensitive one. Clearly some young people do not feel ready to see a doctor on their
own although they may be more comfortable talking to a nurse whom they may
have got to know better through home visits. Staff welcome parental support and
interest but also want to form independent relationships with young people which
are separate from their relationships with the family but not at the expense of them.
They are also wary of overburdening young people with too much responsibility at
too young an age. Some members of staff, many of whom were parents themselves,
admitted that they were not entirely sure how to handle this issue.

I think it's something that I wonder about, because I have a child that's been ill and he's a teenager and I really want to be in there and find out what's going on. He does go to the doctor himself, just because I'm here working, but that experience has made me realise that it might be wrong to expect teenagers to take on as much responsibility as I think we've been expecting them to take on. The evidence is that social support enhances self-management, so I think we should pay more attention to families that we do.
(Diabetes specialist nurse – adult service)

Some mums say, 'I'm not coming in'. Other kids don't want them to interfere but want them to come in with them because they doubt themselves for memorising. I don't know whether we should have a more formal way of letting the child go in and then bringing the parent in afterwards because I think there is – I don't know whether it's our culture – a great need to see them as independent, and that being the all-encompassing thing, this independent person, when really they do need parental support. I think parents often get to a stage when they feel 'Oh right, it's all yours now!' and that really is too much at that age. But if they've had a battle for the last two years, getting them to blood test, getting them to eat properly, they really just think, 'right, you've made these decisions, now you go and face the doctor'.
(Paediatric diabetes specialist nurse)

I try to encourage them to come on their own, certainly to come into the consultation on their own, but that's always been a difficult issue in paediatrics I think. It's always difficult to know quite who the patient is, whether it's the child or whether it's the child and the parent. Obviously it's both, isn't it?
(Consultant paediatrician)

Another reason staff who run adolescent or transition services want young people to begin to consult alone is to prepare them for the adult clinic which they will soon be attending. As they grow to adulthood, nearly all young people will be expected to attend clinic appointments on their own and, in order to make the most of consultations, they should feel confident about talking with professionals, asking questions and making sure they have the advice and information they need.

> It's trying to prepare them for the adult clinic. When they go on to adult services – from what I understand – they're seen by themselves and that's it. It's trying to get a halfway house between having the parents do all the work and leaving them to it themselves.
> *(Paediatric diabetes specialist nurse)*

Although doctors in adult services were prepared for parents accompanying young people to their first appointments at the adult clinic (particularly if transfer was made at a young age as in research area E), they expected to consult with them independently after they had had the opportunity to get to know each other.

> Some may come with mother or father and, if they do, they only bring their parents once, and they subsequently come on their own, which is part of the growing up process.
> *(Consultant physician – adult service)*

One consultant made it clear that he would prefer parents not to be present.

> We've taken the view that as soon as we can get the parents out of the room the better.
> *(Consultant diabetologist – adult service)*

A nurse felt, however, that there should be individual choice about whether or not parents should come into the consultation without pressure imposed either from within or without about what was normal practice.

> I think themselves they feel pressure to come in on their own – often when they get to a particular age they think it looks a bit sissy. And I've occasionally detected from the doctors that they think it's not appropriate for them to be bringing their mummy in but I think that's a very individual thing and I think for a lot of them it's helpful for them to have somebody else there, particularly if they feel intimidated by being sat there with all these health care professionals.
> *(Diabetes specialist nurse – paediatric and adult service)*

A flexible approach that firstly respects the wishes and autonomy of the young person while accommodating parents (and, in some cases, other family members) seems most appropriate. Many adults find attending consultations with doctors intimidating and might want to be accompanied by a partner or friend and this may also be the case with young people. As one paediatrician who runs a joint clinic for young adults with her adult colleagues made clear, the diabetes team should include the young person themselves, their family and friends if they wish and health care professionals.

> Some of the very protective parents … I've already years ago
> started to say well perhaps we should start on our own, as an
> undoing of the apron strings, when they're sort of 13 or
> something. But by the time they get to the young adult clinic
> they can do what they like. I don't think it's for us to start
> saying who can and can't be there. I mean the whole feeling
> is that it's a partnership of trying to look after them of which
> the patient is the main person in charge and we're there for
> advice and help.
> *(Paediatrician)*

Meeting information needs

Another point that was made by staff was the importance of ensuring that young people had the information they need to care for themselves as well as the confidence to use that information. Those who were diagnosed as young children may be less well informed than they should be because they have relied on their parents not only to care for them but to understand diabetes. There is a wealth of information available in the form of leaflets, books, videos and CD-Rom's. Diabetes UK produce magazines, including one aimed at teenagers.

> Probably if they've been diabetic for a number of years as
> children, everything's probably been controlled by their
> parents in a way, and perhaps by the staff at the children's
> hospital.
> *(Diabetes specialist nurse – adult service)*

Information alone is not enough: young people need the confidence to use it. In theory adjusting insulin dose to accommodate different activities and mealtimes may seem straightforward but is more difficult in practice. One paediatrician explained:

> I think the whole team's ethos is to equip the patients to
> make decisions on their own. But not just to give them the
> details, because I think that's not sufficient. What we also
> have to do is to make sure that they are confident enough in
> their knowledge and their ability to make those changes.
> It's all very well thinking you know how to drive a car but if
> you're too scared to get in the driver's seat then you won't
> get very far.
> *(Paediatrician)*

Being well informed can have a direct effect on how a young person might approach looking after themselves. If a young person successfully improves control over a period of three or four months between appointments and this is substantiated by a lower HbA1c result then they can acknowledge and draw confidence from their achievement.

More carrot than stick

If it is hard to get adolescents with 'bulletproof thinking' to take on board the risks of developing complications in adulthood, health care staff may try other approaches to convince young people to improve their control. Younger adolescents may be warned that if they have poor control that they may not grow to their potential height. Some older ones want to learn to drive and will need the signature of a health care professional on the driving licence form. Those members of staff interviewed tried to use incentives that they believed were relevant to the lives of young people.

> Threatening them with anything doesn't work. I think you
> have to make it relevant to what's happening in their life
> now so if the 'Do you want to feel well in yourself?' doesn't
> work, things like, at this age, growing, being as tall as their
> peers, that means you have to have your control good for
> that and things like driving, that's a bit of a carrot, so you
> have to make it relevant.
> *(Paediatric diabetes specialist nurse)*

> There's ways of saying things to them and it's maybe making
> the issues a bit closer to home. Like 'Do you know I have to
> sign a letter for your driving licence?' It might be blackmail
> at the end of the day – hopefully not – but it's bringing it
> down to their level and their life and telling them what they
> can do. And trying to get their control better – not perfect.
> *(Paediatric diabetes specialist nurse)*

Staff also said that sometimes there is a balance to be struck between ensuring
that young people are taking the correct amount of insulin and attending clinic
appointments and expecting the best possible control. For some young people
optimal control may not be possible to achieve because they are not prepared to
test regularly, adjust their insulin accordingly, eat well or take exercise. It is also
harder for some to achieve good control than for others.

> They are not really worried about whether or not you might
> be blind when you are thirty. I think it's important to
> mention complications but I think you're wasting your time
> probably. What they have to concentrate on is to make sure
> that they are taking their insulin and that their health is as
> good as it can be and to know that there are some penalties
> to pay if things don't go well for them so I think it is
> important to point that out but I think overstressing it is
> probably counter-productive.
> *(Consultant diabetologist – adult service)*

> We don't threaten, we do not threaten, not at all. We may
> explain to them the reasons why we would want them to
> have better control, but I would probably go for the tack
> that it would make them feel better first of all rather than
> what it might do for you in 10 or 15 years down the line.
> *(Dietician – adult service)*

> I think as an adolescent, they are old enough usually to
> appreciate what we're talking about and I think it's only fair
> that they know that the reason we want them to have good
> control is for them to avoid problems in the future, and I
> think it would be unfair of me to not tell them so that if they
> were 25 and had eye disease or renal disease they should not
> be able to say no one told me that if I didn't look after

myself that this would happen. So it's a fine line and
sometimes I think we probably get it wrong. We try
desperately to make sure we won't, but it's hard.
(Paediatrician)

Clearly staff feel that achieving good glycaemic control is possible for young
people and that it can be achieved without making too many sacrifices.
However, living with diabetes daily is not easy. Young people must remember to
carry their equipment with them, blood test regularly and be constantly aware
of how their activities affect their control. One respondent who filled in the
quality of life questionnaire expressed her frustration with the condition and
with medical staff.

I have had diabetes for 13 years and I think it is about time
someone found something better than injections. I also
think that medical people don't understand how difficult it
is and will never know unless they have diabetes themselves.
(17 year old female)

Older and wiser

A number of doctors and nurses talked about young people who had poor
control and were irregular clinic attenders during adolescence coming back to
seek out services as young adults.

We try and help them to take more control over it
themselves and that can be a very long process because
everyone's at a different stage and it takes some people
longer to mature than others. We try to introduce more
health issues to them, you know? We wouldn't ram that
down their throat initially but over time we would chip away
at their thinking about later life. But often teenagers'
agendas are quite different and you have to allow for that –
you just have to allow them to take their own time to
mature. And sometimes they're in their mid-twenties before
they really discover what would be best for them.
(Dietician – adult service)

Very often there's a sort of lapse period and then suddenly when they start getting out into the big wide world they think there might be some benefit in looking after themselves.
(Consultant diabetologist – adult service)

There's a small group who [the paediatrician] will always moan that they've been dreadful as 10, 12, 14 year olds and once they leave home or begin to look after themselves, they actually change, improve. Their whole attitude improves, but that's again the growing up process, isn't it?
(Consultant diabetologist – adult service)

These young people have reached an age when they realise the importance of diabetes care. This may be because they are going to university, or have graduated, have started a new relationship, or a first job. One dietician, however, admitted that she did not know exactly what motivated them to change their attitudes or behaviour.

I think it's all about habits actually. So if you can get them in the groove of good habits and then really encourage and support them, I think you're onto a winner. But I'd love to know what pushes the switch, what makes people all of a sudden turn the corner, and there are plenty that do, and when you ask them 'Why have you got so much better?', they say, 'I don't know'.
(Paediatric dietician)

A consultant in the adult service had some suggestions:

I think it's almost more a matter a life events in a way. It might be being admitted to intensive care that gives people the kick up the backside they need and think, 'I nearly died so perhaps I better take this seriously'. In women there's no doubt that pregnancy makes them take their diabetes very seriously … Certain people come back at all sorts of stages of their lives and people will turn up even after sort of two or three years of absence from the clinic and you can look at their HBA1c's and say 'for the last ten years your diabetes has been awful' and they say 'yeah but I've realised that but

> I thought I better change before I get problems' and
> something has made them wake up to it … So everybody
> seems to respond differently – I don't think there is a type
> as such.
> *(Consultant diabetologist – adult service)*

It is important that staff keep young people engaged and encourage them to
attend appointments in the hope that those whose control has been poor will
begin to improve their self-care. The concern is that if they lose contact with
services it will be more difficult to seek care when they are ready to do so as they
will have to return to their GP to be re-referred and will no longer have
personal contact with specialist service providers.

> I think we've probably got to jolly them along and keep
> them on board so that when they become a bit more
> responsible and a bit less risk taking then they're actually
> still in the service so I would try not to nag too much really.
> *(Consultant paediatrician)*

A nurse talked about the dilemma she faces in trying to maintain contact with
young people who have poor control in order to ensure that they are not
storing up problems for the future.

> I'm not very happy with this because I'm basically saying,
> 'Let's put up with less than good sugar levels here for the
> sake of keeping this person coming' because, working in the
> adult sphere as well, I see what happens when they drop out.
> I've got a number of 30-something year old young men
> particularly who have had diabetes since childhood,
> dropped out of care, weren't particularly rigorously followed
> up and have a lot of complications already, and they've just
> started having families and they're looking at renal failure
> and losing vision if they don't have the heart attack that sees
> them off first, you know, and that's in young life. So it is
> difficult. I think it's a huge dilemma really.
> *(Diabetes specialist nurse – paediatric and adult services)*

'I can't live their lives for them'

Despite the commitment of staff members to educating and empowering the young people in their care, they admitted that young people themselves (and their parents or carers) are central to making the difference between good and poor glycaemic control and therefore for health risks they may run. Exactly what makes some young people take on the responsibility for self-care and others fight it is not clear, although the level of support they receive from their families is certainly a factor. Staff talked about how, despite their best efforts, it is down to young people to look after themselves because of the nature of diabetes.

> At the end of the day I think it is the individual who decides to get their act together and I am not sure just how much we influence their outcome. We still have the responsibility and we still have to be here but I think it is the individual patient that is the person who influences how well controlled they are more than anybody else.
> *(Diabetes specialist nurse – adult service)*

> I can't live their lives for them. I'm there, I'm supposed to guide them along in the right direction but, as soon as they're out the door, they're responsible. I can point them in the right direction but I can't give the insulin for them, I can't do their blood testing for them, I can't do their shopping and plan their diet for them.
> *(Consultant diabetologist – adult service)*

8.   Relationships with health care staff

Hospital staff described the philosophies and practices they adopt when caring for young people with diabetes in the previous chapter. Interviews with them show how critical good communication with young people is for effective treatment, as is an understanding of the shared nature of diabetes care across both the multidisciplinary team and the young person and their parents or carers. From young people's perspectives, interaction with staff is probably a more important element of their care than the structural arrangements of their diabetes service. The informality and friendliness of young people's dealings with diabetes specialist nurses, for example, were appreciated by many of those who were interviewed.

The young people who participated in the study were asked about their relationships with staff, answering questions on how well they felt they know health care staff and the quality of those relationships. The significant members of the team for nearly all young people who were interviewed were the doctor (paediatrician or adult physician) and the diabetes specialist nurse or nurses. Dieticians were also mentioned as important. The responses of young people show that, on the whole, the efforts of members of staff are paying off in the sense that their patients are satisfied with the way they are treated. However, a few members of staff, particularly doctors, did come in for criticism.

The quality of relationships with members of the health care team is a principal element of treatment for patients more widely. A systematic literature review on patients' priorities for what constitutes good care in general practice was carried out as part of a project by the European Task Force on Patient Evaluations of General Practice (Coulter 2002). It showed that 'humaneness' is the most highly rated aspect of care, followed by 'competence', 'patients' involvement in decisions' and 'time for care'. In the current study, young people were asked to rate how well they knew their doctor, nurse, dietician and other health care staff they had contact with and to answer questions about what made these relationships successful or not. All the aspects of care referred to above were mentioned by young respondents in assessing what characterises good relationships with staff. They clearly appreciated the 'humaneness' and 'time for care' offered in particular by diabetes specialist nurses, the 'competence' of doctors and nurses and the opportunity to be involved in decision making about their care.

What young people said about health care staff

More than half of the young people interviewed (53 per cent) said they felt that they knew the doctor who treated them 'very well' or 'quite well' (Table 8.1). Those who attended paediatric or transition clinics (where they were still in contact with paediatricians) were more likely to say they knew the doctor well (73 per cent) compared to those who attended adult clinics (33 per cent). In line with this finding there were more respondents who attended adult clinics who knew the doctor only 'a bit' or 'not at all'. This is not surprising as many young people will have been treated by the same paediatrician for some years whereas those who attend adult clinics, where appointments are less frequent, may have met the doctor only once or twice.

Table 8.1 How well do you know the doctor?

	n	%
Very well	10	12
Quite well	35	41
A bit	21	25
Not at all	16	19
Do not see a doctor	3	3
Total	85	100

Young people were also asked how well they knew the diabetes specialist nurse, dietician and other members of staff. The results for nurses and dieticians are reported in Tables 8.2 and 8.3. So few respondents felt that they knew podiatrists, optometrists or psychologists that the results of questions concerning these disciplines have not been included.

Table 8.2 How well do you know the nurse?

	n	%
Very well	30	35
Quite well	24	28
A bit	15	18
Not at all	11	13
Do not see a nurse	5	6
Total	85	100

As can be seen from Tables 8.1 and 8.2, a higher proportion of respondents said they knew the diabetes specialist nurse 'very well' or 'quite well' (63 per cent) compared with the doctor (53 per cent). Qualitative data from the interviews explains why young people feel they know nurses better. They are more likely to have contact with a nurse between appointments, receive a home visit from a nurse and have time to talk informally with a nurse at clinic appointments. Young people described the role of the diabetes specialist nurses as more social and less medical than that of doctors whom they usually see in the formal context of a hospital consultation.

> She is easier to talk to and she is always available whenever
> I ring up.
> *(18 year old female)*

> Well they [nurse and dietician] were the ones that came
> to my house and they were kind of cool.
> *(16 year old female)*

> I think [the doctor] is in charge and she is giving you more
> formal advice than [the nurse]. [The nurse] will then put
> things into context, if you see what I mean. I can't really think
> of examples. [The nurse] is less medical, more real life.
> *(17 year old female)*

More than 40 per cent of respondents did not see a dietician with any regularity although they had had dietetic advice when they were first diagnosed. Only 18 per cent felt they knew a dietician well and nearly 40 per cent 'a bit' or 'not at all'. In one of the hospitals the dietician was also the diabetes team manager and played an active role both in the clinic and between appointments. Six of the respondents who said they knew a dietician well were patients at that hospital.

Table 8.3 How well do you know the dietician?

	n	%
Very well	3	4
Quite well	12	14
A bit	13	15
Not at all	20	23
Do not see a dietician	37	44
Total	85	100

Of those who felt they knew a doctor well enough to comment on the way they were treated, the large majority found doctors 'always' or 'usually' respectful, understanding and supportive (Table 8.4). However, over 10 per cent felt they were not treated with 'understanding' and nearly a third (31 per cent) said that doctors could be patronising. The numbers of respondents in these categories are small but their experience of not being treated kindly or with respect show that a minority of doctors have not gained the trust of their young patients. While a few young people felt that doctors were critical in a bullying way, others mentioned helpful and constructive criticism which they were more inclined to accept and act upon.

Table 8.4 What is the doctor like?

Is the doctor…	respectful?		understanding?		supportive?		patronising?		critical?		does the doctor listen?	
	n	%	n	%	n	%	n	%	n	%	n	%
Always	54	73	47	64	49	66	5	7	5	7	51	69
Usually	12	16	18	24	17	23	2	3	6	8	17	23
Sometimes	5	7	6	8	6	8	16	21	28	38	4	5
Never	3	4	3	4	2	3	51	69	35	47	2	3
Total	74	100	74	100	74	100	74	100	74	100	74	100

Only 74 respondents felt they knew a doctor well enough to answer these questions

In terms of their relationships with diabetes specialist nurses, young people were more positive. None of the respondents was in contact with a nurse who was never respectful, understanding or supportive or who never listened to them (Table 8.5). As with doctors, some young people said nurses were critical but that the criticism was welcomed if constructive and non-judgemental.

Table 8.5 What is the nurse like?

Is the nurse…	respectful?		understanding?		supportive?		patronising?		critical?		does the nurse listen?	
	n	%	n	%	n	%	n	%	n	%	n	%
Always	58	92	55	87	57	91	1	2	1	2	59	94
Usually	5	8	7	11	4	6	2	3	4	6	4	6
Sometimes			1	2	2	3	4	6	17	27		
Never							56	89	41	65		
Total	63	100	63	100	63	100	63	100	63	100	63	100

Only 63 respondents felt they knew a nurse well enough to answer these questions

Only 14 young people felt they knew a dietician well enough to comment on how they treated them and, therefore, this data has not been reported.

As shown in Table 8.6, most young people felt they had a 'very good' or 'quite good' relationship with the doctor (88 per cent) and a larger proportion of those who answered this question felt their relationship with the nurse was good (98 per cent). All those who responded to this question about dieticians felt they had a good relationship (although the numbers are small in this category).

Table 8.6 Relationships with hospital staff

Do you have a good relationship with…	the doctor?		the nurse?		the dietician?	
	n	%	n	%	n	%
Very good	34	46	40	63	7	50
Quite good	31	42	22	35	7	50
Not really	5	6	1	2		
No	2	3				
Don't know	2	3				
Total	74	100	63	100	14	100

More than half (53 per cent) of the 83 young people who answered said their best relationship was with a specialist nurse (Table 8.7).

Table 8.7 Which member of staff do you have the best relationship with?

	n	%
Doctor	22	27
Nurse	44	53
Doctor and nurse equally	7	8
Dietician	2	2
Not sure	8	10
Total	83	100

Two respondents did not answer this question

As noted above, young people felt that their relationships with nurses were less formal than those with doctors and that these relationships were more like those they had with friends or family. They felt able to talk about things that were not directly associated with diabetes and this was reciprocated by nurses who sometimes talked about their own lives. Young people also valued the 'time for care' that nurses had to talk informally with them.

> I mean the thing I like about her is she chats to you. It feels like you're talking normally rather than talking about my diabetes. She's quite understanding of people of my age – the kinds of things we do and how it affects the diabetes.
> *(17 year old female)*

> We can have a laugh. She's a good listener. I can talk to her. She don't boss me.
> *(17 year old male)*

> She's funny and she's all the things you like about people.
> *(10 year old female)*

> She's there for you and gives you information.
> *(17 year old female)*

> I think it's because I've got to know her better as a person, it's not just someone that I go into the clinic to see. I'm sure the others would be just as approachable but, as I say, she's got more time to spend talking to me if I need to.
> *(20 year old female)*

Continuity of care made a difference to how comfortable young people felt with staff members. Some explained that having known a nurse since being diagnosed with diabetes made them feel especially cared for.

> I've always had a nice relationship with her. She can be like a friend to me sometimes, and I've always got on really well with her. She was the first one that come to see me when I was first diabetic and she got me doing my finger pricks and things like that. She's always been there. Whatever I do she listens to me. If it's a thing not about diabetes, she'll sit and listen, she's just really caring and really nice and supportive.
> *(16 year old female)*

> She's friendly and supportive and she visited the house before and things. When I first became diabetic she was always there for me.
> *(15 year old female)*

Discontinuity of care was described as frustrating by one 18 year old male.

> I have a different doctor each time I go so I don't know them at all. That's the main thing that really gets to me is that I go in and there's a different doctor every time and you have to start from … there was one doctor and I went in and she started explaining how diabetes works and I said, 'Look I've been a diabetic for seven years, listen, I know that. That's not what I want to be told.' I walked out of that one. I just walked straight out – I couldn't hack it. She was talking like I was, you know, a nursery kid or summat, and I was like 'flippin' 'eck'. I just walked straight out.

Another explained how he found it difficult talking to people he does not know and the effect staff leaving has on him.

> It takes me a little while. I don't usually open up to people but, I mean, because the last few doctors I've had have left, I have got to know them really well and I talked to them even outside of the centre but they are all leaving and I am just afraid that they are going to leave again so that is why I don't usually open up that much any more. I can usually talk more to the nurses because they are usually there for a little bit longer.
> *(16 year old male)*

Although more young people said they had the 'best' relationship with a nurse, a larger proportion said that doctors were the most important member of staff in helping them manage diabetes although eight individuals thought it was a combination of both the doctor and nurse (Table 8.8).

Table 8.8 Which member of staff is most important in helping you manage diabetes?

	n	%
Doctor	38	45
Nurse	30	36
Doctor and nurse equally	8	9
Dietician	2	3
Not sure	6	7
Total	84	100

One respondent did not answer this question

From the interviews with young people, it seems that they expect to have different relationships with doctors and nurses. Although they value the informality of their relationships with nurses and the support they receive from them, they understand that the doctor is the person who will advise them about their insulin dose and talk to them about screening results and they recognise that the doctor has more power to make clinical decisions.

> [The doctor] will say 'You need to up your insulin' or things like that. I think he'll be the one who makes those decisions.
> *(17 year old female)*

> If there's anything that I really need to talk to someone about there's really not much point in talking to [the nurse] 'cause she'll just tell me to talk to [the doctor].
> *(18 year old female)*

> [The doctor's] the one who has helped me to understand diabetes so that makes me know more about it and know how I should be treating it. She puts things into perspective and a life context so you can actually make sense of it. She's quite good like that.
> *(17 year old female)*

However, young people may not expect to have a rapport with the doctor. Some found doctors less approachable than nurses and sometimes difficult to talk to – and to understand.

> I think he's very fair, he tries to sort of get it over to you, doesn't he? That's all he's trying to do, but she thinks he's trying to catch her out all the time. I think he's nice.
> *(mother of 17 year old female)*

> I mean [the doctor] is, I dunno, he's quite an old guy, well, he's not really old. Just seems like a typical doctor that will frown upon you if you tell him anything whereas [the nurse], if you tell her that you went out and got drunk the night before and you weren't feeling too bad, she would take it in a different way and she wouldn't make you feel bad about it, you know, so I think [the nurse] is much better to talk to about those sort of things and sometimes when I'm there and he asks me a question, I'll be in two minds whether to tell him because I'll get a lecture about what I've said.
> *(19 year old male)*

> He knows what he is on about but he doesn't like sort of say it in terms that you know. He will tell me something and I haven't got a clue what he is talking about.
> *(16 year old male)*

Young people's responses to the questions about relationships with staff showed that they were, on the whole, happy with the way they were treated. More felt comfortable talking to nurses than to doctors but they were aware of the importance of the doctor in helping them manage diabetes. Some doctors were popular with young patients but some did not seem able to communicate on their wavelength and could perhaps build more trusting relationships if they behaved more like nurses. One young man, for example, suggested that doctors would benefit from the qualities a nurse brought to her role.

> I think [the nurse] would have been a really cracking doctor, you know, someone like her who's a doctor would be ace.
> *(19 year old male)*

9.   Living with diabetes

This study concentrated on the health care young people with diabetes experience in hospital clinics. However, young people themselves are fundamental to their own care as they are the ones who have to manage diabetes on a daily basis. Young people's family and social worlds are also important for both their physical and psychological health as they are for all young people. Participants in the study were asked to comment on the level and quality of support offered by family members, friends and members of staff in schools, colleges and workplaces. Parents and other family members were not interviewed although, in some cases, parents and/or siblings sat in on or participated in interviews.

Who is important?

Self-management is an essential aspect of diabetes care. The person with diabetes has to manage the condition on a daily basis, controlling diet, insulin dose and exercise and testing blood regularly. Although health care staff offer medical advice and treatment, the young person is usually the main carer. Family and friends are also likely to be available for support between clinic appointments. In order to ascertain to what extent young people felt they were in control of caring for themselves, they were asked who they considered was important in managing diabetes (Table 9.1).

The large majority (93 per cent) felt that they themselves were 'very important' in managing diabetes while 6 per cent thought they were 'quite important' and only one individual thought they were 'not important'. Depending on their age, the length of time that they had had diabetes and their level of independence, young people viewed themselves, family, friends and health care staff as more or less central to their care.

Table 9.1 Who is important in managing diabetes?

	You		Family		Hospital staff		GP		Friends	
	n	%	n	%	n	%	n	%	n	%
Very important	79	93	38	45	33	39	6	7	10	12
Quite important	5	6	41	48	42	49	24	28	45	53
Not important	1	1	6	7	10	12	55	65	30	35
Total	85	100	85	100	85	100	85	100	85	100

Of the 42 young people who had not yet moved to adult care, for example, 50 per cent still considered their family to be 'very important' compared to 39 per cent of those in adult care. Of those 43 who were attending adult clinics, 51 per cent thought their families were 'quite important' to their care compared to 48 per cent of those who had not yet transferred to adult care. Five of those who had transferred to adult care did not consider their family to be important in managing diabetes (these five had all left home) compared to only one of those not yet in adult care. More than half of both groups, however, said that one of their parents, in most cases their mother, took responsibility for making sure that they attended clinic appointments. Nearly three-quarters of those who had not transferred to adult care thought that their friends were important in managing diabetes compared to 60 per cent of those in adult care.

Hospital staff were considered 'very' or 'quite' important by 90 per cent of those not yet in adult care and by 86 per cent of those in adult care. Ten young people did not think that hospital staff were important to their care. GPs were seen by the majority (60 per cent of both groups) as not being important. Young people did not see their GP for diabetes care but do get prescriptions from the GP.

Family support for young people with diabetes

Previous studies on the interactions between diabetes and family life have focused on family types, family stress and their effect on self-care and on glycaemic control, usually measured by HbA1c levels (Hanson *et al.* 1987, Marteau *et al.* 1987, Viner *et al.* 1996). They provide evidence of the importance of the family to adolescents living with diabetes as well as the consequences of family stress. Research has shown that better glycaemic control is associated with families who maintain involvement in adolescents' diabetes care (Follansbee 1989, Grey *et al.* 1998). One of the health care workers interviewed for the study believed that, similarly, poor control is linked to social or psychological problems.

> It might not be something that people would generally think of as a social problem ... It might be something like the teenager doesn't want to tell the new boyfriend that they've got diabetes, or it might be that they're getting called a drug addict because they use a pen to give their insulin, so it might not be what people typically think of as a social or psychological issue but to me there's always something like that at the root of poor control.
> *(Paediatric dietician)*

Other studies have considered the effects of peer support in relation to adolescents' self-care and quality of life (La Greca *et al.* 1995b, Olsen and Sutton 1998, Skinner and Hampson 1998). As young people grow increasingly independent of their parents, they spend more time with others of their own age. Olsen and Sutton found that the adolescents they interviewed had differing views about independence and privacy and this affected how they wanted their friends to behave in relation to diabetes. Some preferred friends not to mention diabetes and not to comment on their behaviour, while others liked to be reminded that their friends cared about them. La Greca *et al.* (1995b) investigated the different levels and kinds of support offered by family members and friends to young people with diabetes. They found that support from family members, particularly parents, was primarily 'tangible' support, while friends offered 'companionship' and 'emotional' support. 'Tangible' support was defined as tasks involved in overseeing a young person's day to day management of diabetes. These included reminding adolescents about what they need to do on a daily basis, taking insulin and blood testing, for example, and making sure they had everything they needed when they leave the house as well as providing appropriate meals, picking up prescriptions and accompanying them to clinic appointments. Family members also shared lifestyle tasks with young people by eating the same kinds of food, exercising together and, in some cases, doing insulin injections for them.

Data from the interviews with young people in this study showed that they valued the support they received from parents. Some felt that their parents had been overprotective towards them, especially in the period after diagnosis of diabetes, but they understood the concerns of parents and other family members and some admitted that they liked the attention. They described the 'tangible' support offered by family members and also the 'emotional' support they received from both family and friends as well as the concern that parents felt for their well-being. Many appreciated the fact that their parents were increasingly allowing them to take responsibility for their own care and were relieved that parents worried less as they grew older and had been living with diabetes for longer. None of the young people interviewed said that their parents had not supported them or felt that they would have liked more support. One young woman, whose parents had moved to another part of the country, felt her self-care and clinic attendance had deteriorated after the move but said that her mother still rang to remind her to go to clinic appointments. University students living away from home also reported that their parents were still involved in their care by supportive telephone calls and reminders about clinic attendance. A number of students returned to their home town to stay with their parents and attend hospital appointments there.

Young people's comments about the support they received from family members, especially parents, are a reminder that diabetes is something that must be dealt with continually. Much of the day to day support parents offer acts as a reminder to young people about carrying equipment with them as well as making sure they are eating well and at the right times. Parents' input is particularly important when young people are ill.

> They make sure I've got everything I need and, I mean, they always make sure I've got my blood test kit and my injections – I'd probably forget it otherwise.
> *(15 year old male)*

> Me mum is always bringing me up my breakfast in bed in the morning so that I eat and get food inside me for when I get the injection done. She's always making sure if we go out that I have got my stuff with me and my blood kit. My dad every morning before he goes to work makes me do a blood test. They monitor my blood more than I do really.
> *(19 year old female)*

> They shout at me when I ain't done blood tests and tell me
> to do my injections.
> *(17 year old male)*

> My mum is like 'make sure you've got your injections' about
> ten times. I say 'yes, Mum, I've got my injections and I've got
> a sweet. Just in case!'
> *(15 year old female)*

> They help me do my injections and they get all my insulins
> from like the doctors and stuff.
> *(16 year old male)*

> They help me work out my dosages and things if they need
> changing.
> *(16 year old male)*

> My mum helps if I have hypos in the night.
> *(20 year old female)*

> I get a bollocking if I don't do my injections and stuff like that.
> *(18 year old male)*

Young people also reported that siblings were involved in supporting them.

> My brothers and sister are younger than me but they all
> got told and had to learn exactly what to do when I ran low
> … I think they liked it because I had this new machine and
> I could test the levels of blood sugar and see how abnormal
> we all were!
> *(21 year old female)*

Four participants described how family members had changed their diet in
order to support the child with diabetes. Siblings were also expected to adapt to
the new regime.

> My brother is older but we are very close age wise so back in
> the days when Mum used to weigh everything, he would get
> the same sort of portions so it would be easier for my mum
> to work it out.
> *(20 year old male)*

> As soon as I got it, everything was changed in the house. Food was adapted and everyone adapted their diet to suit me … All the drinks now in our house are always diet or sugar-free.
> *(21 year old female)*

> They all kind of eat the same food now. With no sweets in the house because I can't eat them.
> *(17 year old female)*

> My mum helps with my meals, making sure I've got the right food and that in the house.
> *(20 year old female)*

Young people also appreciated that their parents were well informed about diabetes.

> I mean they're really good with it and my mum knows exactly how it works. She looks into it in great detail and so she's a great help.
> *(19 year old female)*

> My mum is always reading extra material about diabetes and new things that are coming out and treatments.
> *(18 year old female)*

They also recognised that parents accepted their growing maturity by giving them space to be independent and allow them to look after themselves.

> When I first was diabetic she [mother] was really over-protective. She was making sure I was doing my blood tests, watching me while I did my blood tests and my insulin to make sure I was getting it right. I felt then that she was overprotective. She just leaves me to get on with it now. Occasionally she says, 'I hope you're still doing your blood tests'.
> *(16 year old female)*

> Maybe my parents were a little overprotective to start with because it was very much new territory for all of us but when it started to settle down, they got used to it and I got used to it at the same time really.
> *(22 year old male)*

They give me independence but I know that they are always there if I need to talk to them about it.
(18 year old female)

I'm happy with how they act because they do try and let me get on with it. They just like to make sure that I'm keeping up with it all.
(17 year old female)

They don't really have much to do with it anymore because I think they know I can deal with it myself. I've been diabetic for nearly seven years now so … If I needed help they would be fine.
(18 year old female)

My mum's been quite good really – in fact everyone has. They've always kind of left me to my own devices. If I have a problem I sort it out. They don't kind of mollycoddle me that much. I don't rely on anyone else.
(22 year old male)

Three young people, however, felt that their parents were overprotective even when, in their view, it was no longer necessary. They contrasted parental expectations of their behaviour with that of their siblings.

It does my head in really 'cause Mum and Dad let go of [my brother and sister] at quite a young age but as soon as I got diabetes it was like going back to square one and now it's always, even at my age, 'Have you done your insulin? Done your bloods? Do this, do that' and I'm, like, give it a rest, you know. I feel like being Kevin from Harry Enfield. 'Leave me alone. Please.' I feel in that respect they're still mothering me too much.
(21 year old male)

Things like I've noticed like when I first went out drinking. How protective they are still if I am going out for the night. 'Have you got this? Have you got that?', whereas my brother can just go and 'We'll see you on such and such a day'. My brother and I go out on our own and whether it's because I'm female or whether it's because of my diabetes, I don't know.
(21 year old female)

> They just worry more when I go out … They go a bit
> overboard I think.
> *(19 year old male)*

However, one young man said he would be sorry if his parents were not worried about him.

> Sometimes it [parents' protectiveness] annoys me but
> they're all just so worried. I would be angry if they weren't!
> *(17 year old male)*

Two others mentioned the emotional support they received from parents, particularly at times when life with diabetes is a struggle.

> I get a lot of support from my mum. If I have my off days,
> feeling down because of my diabetes, depressed … she's
> always there for me to talk to.
> *(16 year old female)*

> My dad was always there for me. Like if he could have it and
> not me then for sure he'd have it and he still says that
> actually to this day.
> *(19 year old female)*

The interviews with young people show their growing independence and the increasing importance of self-management of diabetes as they grow older. However, parental support acts as a reinforcement to self-care. Parents who remind young people to take necessary equipment with them, provide healthy meals, pick up insulin supplies and drive their children to clinic appointments but who still allow them a degree of autonomy are backing up young people's efforts to take responsibility for their own care.

Support from friends

Young people were also asked if their friends supported them and, if so, in what ways. They mentioned 'tangible' support, meaning that friends knew what to do if they become hypoglycaemic and nagged them if they ate too many sweet things or drank too much alcohol. Sometimes friends were able to spot the signs of a hypo before the young person with diabetes. However, young people felt they needed little active support from friends on a day to day basis and did not mention needing or receiving emotional support from friends except in the sense that they appreciated not being treated differently from others while being aware that their friends were well informed enough to look after them if necessary. Despite valuing their independence, most young people were reassured that their friends took an interest in diabetes and were prepared to look after them if necessary. None of them said they needed to talk to friends about the difficulties of living with diabetes but friends did provide 'companionship support' (La Greca *et al.* 1995b) by being 'diabetes aware' and hence prepared to make accommodations for their friend's needs in terms of meals, arrangements for going out and, in some cases, accompanying their friend to the diabetes clinic.

> I have great friends. They know what time I have to eat so when we go out, we go out early even though they eat later.
> *(17 year old male)*

> They're always asking me, 'are you all right?' if I'm a bit low and they say 'are you having one of your hypos?' and I say 'yeah' and they probably buy me a sweet or something.
> *(16 year old male)*

> I've had hypos a couple of times at school and my mates have known what to do. They've got me a can of Coke and made me drink that until they've been able to get me some sugar and that.
> *(16 year old female)*

> I've had one or two hypos when I'm out with my friends. If no one's in the house, they get me front door keys and get me something to eat. Someone will probably stay with me just to make sure I don't have another funny turn.
> *(17 year old male)*

> My best mates or my girlfriend, because I'm around them the most, they're the ones that notice when I'm low or if I'm high or whatever because they can just see it in my face so they tell me if I'm not realising because I usually tell them I'm just going to have a Mars bar or whatever.
> *(16 year old male)*

However, a minority of those interviewed were sometimes irritated by friends who thought they could spot the symptoms of hypoglycaemia. Someone with diabetes can be 'moody' even if they are not suffering from a hypo!

> Some of my friends are really great. They'll even know by my behaviour when I'm low or high … It's just when people I know say, if I get in a bad mood and it's not related to diabetes, then they say, 'do a jab' or 'have some sugar' and there's nothing more annoying than that really.
> *(21 year old male)*

Friends may take on a protective role.

> They always keep an eye on me. Make sure I'm not doing anything too stupid. I always tell them that I've got my phone on me. If any hassles, just dial two and get straight through to my mother or three to get to my sister.
> *(22 year old male)*

> They are quite supportive to me and stuff and, when they find I have had too many sweet things, they will then tell me that I shouldn't be having them and things like that.
> *(15 year old female)*

> They watch out for me. 'You shouldn't be eating that!'
> *(15 year old female)*

Two young people described not wanting to tell people about having diabetes because they feel uncomfortable about mentioning it or do not want to be identified primarily as someone with diabetes.

> I am a bit shy, I don't like to tell. I think I get embarrassed about it.
> *(15 year old female)*

> People I meet, they probably find out a few months down the line that I've got it. It's not something I say. Unless they catch me and I'm on a hypo or something and they're like 'what's wrong with you?' and I'm like, 'give me a biscuit'.
> *(19 year old female)*

Two young people did not feel they needed support from friends and that friends were ignorant about diabetes. These young men had not educated their friends about diabetes and did not seem to think it was necessary or helpful to do so.

> They don't really understand what it means. For instance, some of them think that you get diabetes from eating too much sugar and stuff like that. They don't understand it at all. They are neither here nor there really. They just know I've got it and that's about it.
> *(20 year old male)*

> It's not an issue really. I can't actually remember a situation when I've ever needed help from any of my friends, you know, had problems with my diabetes. I know they know I've got diabetes but they don't really know what it is or anything. It's just like I have to inject myself basically. That's all they know.
> *(18 year old male)*

One young man, who was diagnosed with diabetes at the age of four, said:

> They don't really have anything to do with it. They know but it doesn't really affect them. I haven't known any different.
> *(23 year old male)*

Some of those interviewed mentioned peers who they felt were thoughtless or unkind because they had diabetes.

> The only thing that annoys me is if a mate of mine phones me up and says 'What are you doing? Let's go out' and I say, 'Well look I've got to have dinner now'. So I have to miss out occasionally.
> *(17 year old male)*

> Yeah, my friends are all right about it. A couple of them know. A couple of them don't really want to know.
> *(17 year old male)*

> I just keep it quiet. Some people take the mickey out of it. They say horrible things and that.
> *(10 year old female)*

Most of the young people interviewed appreciated the fact that friends accommodated their diabetes as part of their relationships although the nature of this accommodation was individualised in the sense that some wanted and accepted emotional support while others were more private about having diabetes and preferred friends to make little of it. Because coping with diabetes is something that young people have to do all the time, they need friends who can support them in the ways that they find comfortable and this may mean rejecting people who are unable or unwilling to offer that support. One young man, who had been hospitalised with DKA on a number of occasions, had stopped seeing friends who had not been prepared to accommodate his diabetes because he felt they were a bad influence on him, particularly during a period when he was finding it difficult to accept what he saw as the constraints of living with diabetes.

> When I first got diagnosed with it [aged 14], I was finding it harder because I always wanted to be out with my mates and then I was having to come in at half five to do my injections, stay in for half an hour and have something to eat whereas normally I would stay out and play football with my mates all the time or just do like what normal teenagers do. I don't hang around with them people no more because when I was hanging around them I weren't looking after myself.
> *(18 year old male)*

Another was clear that friends had to accept him as he is.

> Girlfriends, most of them have been fine. Sometimes maybe a bit of a shock to start with when they see me pulling out needles and testing my blood all the time but, if they're not happy with it, that's their own problem. They can take a hike. It comes as a package really. It's not as if I can get rid of it.
> *(23 year old male)*

Living with diabetes at school

There is evidence that young people with medical needs may not get the support they need from school staff, particularly in secondary schools. Previous studies have highlighted teachers' lack of knowledge about diabetes and parents' dissatisfaction with schools' care of their child's diabetes (Burden *et al.*

1990, Tatman and Lessing 1993, Bolton 1997, Branson and Ellerby 1997). Despite guidance from the government (DfEE 1996), some young people with medical needs have experienced discrimination because school staff are unwilling to involve them in all activities (Lightfoot *et al.* 2001). The highly publicised case of a boy with diabetes who was not allowed to go on a school trip drew attention to the fact that school policy is not always inclusive. The Special Educational Needs and Disability Act 2001, which came into force in September 2002, should go some way to ensuring that schools develop policies to prevent pupils with disabilities (which include chronic conditions such as diabetes) being treated less favourably than other children. Schools' duties under the Act cover 'education and associated services' which include teaching, learning, lunch breaks, school policies, exam arrangements, timetabling and school trips and journeys (Stobbs 2001).

Young people who were interviewed as part of the current study were asked whether and in what ways staff at school, university and work supported them. Their answers point to a mixed picture. Some reported that staff were well informed and supportive, while others said that staff were ignorant about diabetes and felt that their friends were better able to look after them if they needed help. In some cases, teachers had visited young people in hospital when they were first diagnosed and made sure that pupils were supported when they returned to school, while other young people reported that teachers were unwilling to take the time to understand the needs of a pupil with diabetes.

> All of them know and they always make sure I'm all right
> and that and the nurse sometimes makes sure I'm all right
> and that when she's in.
> *(16 year old male)*

> That's one criticism I've got. They've [school staff] got no
> idea. The nurse is in one day a week. And they don't have
> like trained First Aid people which is like astonishing.
> They're certainly not as up to speed with things as they
> should be.
> *(Mother of 16 year old male)*

Parents had a role to play in explaining their children's needs to school staff and, in some cases, acted as advocate on behalf of a child who was being bullied because of having diabetes.

At primary school my mum went to see the headmaster – I think I was about six – and told him I had diabetes and the headmaster was saying, 'oh, I don't think you can stay at this school. You'll have to go to a special school.' Mum got upset.
(16 year old male)

He had a very good teacher at primary school who went up to the hospital when he was first ill. I did go there and explain to them how to do things if he thought he was going into hypo.
(Mother of 17 year old male)

I had a lot of trouble when I first went to school. Everyone used to call me names and say I was a druggie 'cause I took insulin and my mum supported me through that. She talked to the teachers.
(16 year old female)

The support young people received in schools seemed to depend on individual members of staff who took on the responsibility of being knowledgeable and available. Most young people found someone at school, apart from their friends, whom they would approach if they were hypoglycaemic or unwell. This might be the school secretary, caretaker, nurse or a particular teacher. However, many reported that there was no whole school policy to ensure that all members of staff were aware that a pupil had diabetes, or presumably another chronic condition, and what they needed to know to care for them if they became hypoglycaemic.

When I went to my comprehensive school, I went in the day before I started and I went to see who was going to be my tutor and we sat down and we spoke through it all. She knew exactly what I needed. The support's there I think if you need it.
(19 year old female)

One of my teachers at school is diabetic and that is who I go to … He is really helpful because at school there is not too much awareness of it but with him I just go and he knows how to sort it out.
(16 year old male)

> There is a caretaker there and he is quite nice about it and
> he buys me glucose tablets to have at school in case I go low.
> I think he is a First Aider.
> *(15 year old female)*

> The teachers really didn't know much. It was more like the
> secretary where I went when I knew I was quite bad.
> Sometimes they sent me home if I said I wasn't too good. Or
> sometimes if I didn't have anything that I could take they'd
> get me something from the canteen.
> *(17 year old male)*

> Not a lot of the staff knew about it. It was just a certain one that
> I could go to and I'd get something to eat and that from them.
> *(16 year old female)*

Eating at school

One of the issues mentioned most often by young people was the need to eat between meals. In order to maintain optimal levels, young people with diabetes may need to have a snack if their blood sugar is low or lowering. Leaving a lesson to get a snack or eating in class may be awkward or embarrassing and the attitude of teaching staff can make a difference to how comfortable young people feel. Some of those interviewed said that other pupils made them feel that eating in class was a privilege they had not earned. Clear policies and a well informed lead from teachers could ensure that peers understand more about the medical needs of classmates and would make schools more inclusive for those who may feel 'different'.

Two respondents described negative experiences:

> I had to eat my lunch in class and that was really awful
> because everyone was looking at me. No one was nasty about
> it but, when I sort of started munching away in the middle of
> the history lesson, there were a few looks like, 'why can she
> and can't I?'
> *(17 year old female)*

> I have to go and stand outside all on my own to eat and it
> gets on my nerves and then I walk back in and everyone's
> like 'so out of order – I wish I had it' and I'm like, 'Yeah,
> alright then, try injecting yourself twice a day'.
> *(16 year old female)*

Another pupil was not made to feel uncomfortable:

> They [teachers] all know I'm a diabetic so if I'm in the
> middle of class and I need something to eat and I haven't
> got nothing on me I always just ask and they say, 'yes, it's OK
> if you go out and get yourself something to eat from the
> vending machine'. They don't really mind.
> *(17 year old male)*

Being 'different'

Although there was no wide-ranging reporting of being treated differently by
peers at school, two young people mentioned being bullied by other pupils
when they first went to school. One was called a 'druggie' and the other said,
'I got the mick taken out of me by a couple of girls'. In one case, the pupil's
mother came to the school to talk to staff about it.

Two other respondents mentioned members of school staff who made their lives
difficult although not apparently deliberately. The first attended an
independent boarding school and was not allowed to keep his insulin and
equipment with him which he found frustrating because he had to find the
member of staff who kept it who was based on the other side of the school from
the dining room. Another was angry that his 'teenage' behaviour was associated
by teachers with his having diabetes. He felt this was based on a lack of
understanding, of both him and of diabetes, rather than intentional but was
upset by the fact that his attitude and actions were seen to be determined by
having diabetes.

Communication between health and school staff

There is a case for health care and education staff communicating more often
and more effectively in order to support the inclusion of children with
chronic conditions in mainstream schools (Mukherjee *et al.* 2000, 2002).

One way that this can happen is by diabetes specialist nurses visiting schools to educate school staff about pupils' needs. Young people interviewed for this study were asked whether a nurse had visited their school. Over three-quarters said they had not been visited at school or could not remember a visit (Table 9.2), although two-thirds had been visited at home by a nurse. It is possible, however, that a visit might have been made without the young person's knowledge. In one area there were no reported visits to a school and, in another, only one.

Table 9.2 Has the diabetes specialist nurse visited your school?

	n	%
Yes, more than once	3	4
Yes, once	15	18
No	66	77
Don't remember	1	1
Total	85	100

This information about visits to schools is disappointing since, like all children, those with diabetes spend a large amount of time at school. Diabetes UK recommends an annual school visit for every child and as long ago as 1993 it was suggested that a paediatric diabetes specialist nurse should make school visits and talk to all members of staff who come in contact with the child, including canteen staff and classroom assistants (Tatman and Lessing 1993). However, figures of reported visits were too small in all areas to be meaningfully analysed. Young people, and especially their parents, were reassured by the contact between health care staff and school.

> She [nurse] visited the school. I can't remember how many times, more than once actually. She did a kind of diabetes awareness thing, where she talked about it a bit.
> *(17 year old female)*

> Well, when I first started my middle school, she went in and saw the teachers, but she didn't see me. She just went in and did like a briefing for them.
> *(17 year old male)*

In their study about the communication between health services and school staff, Mukherjee *et al.* (2002) found that the extent to which health professionals communicated with school staff, and the way they went about it, varied widely. Participants in that study recommended the clarification of the roles of health and education staff with regard to children with a chronic illness and of how information should flow from health to school staff. The availability of a school nursing service to both primary and secondary schools is also very variable, as is the nature and scope of the service.

10. Diabetes and quality of life

Diabetes cannot be cured and, until a cure is found, people with type 1 diabetes must regulate their own blood glucose levels for the rest of their lives. As already discussed, the main aim of diabetes management is to control levels so that they are as near as possible to the normal range in order to prevent or postpone the development of complications. Despite recent progress in the manufacture of insulins and of equipment for administering insulin and testing blood which enable people with diabetes to live less rigidly, daily injections, blood tests and monitoring of food intake and exercise are complex and demanding. These tasks of diabetes management may become particularly daunting and difficult to maintain during adolescence and there is clear evidence that there is a worsening of glycaemic control at this time (see, for example, Allen *et al.* 1992).

Increasingly, health service professionals are acknowledging the role of the person living with a chronic illness as being a key member of the care team. As the interviews with staff in this study show, this means that young people with diabetes are asked to share their lifestyle aspirations with staff in order that management can be modelled around them. A second aim, therefore, of diabetes management is to allow the patient to live as 'normal' a life as possible while maintaining and, if necessary, improving blood glucose levels. There is a circular relationship between keeping physically well and feeling good about one's life and the philosophy behind this more holistic approach to treatment is that young people with diabetes who are well informed and take a positive attitude to their condition are likely to be more successful in taking control of their care.

Although intensive diabetes management can improve glycaemic control, it may impair quality of life. Holman and Lorig (2000) argue that 'the goal [of treatment] is not cure but maintenance of pleasurable and independent living'. However, anxieties about future health, feeling 'different' from peers and siblings, family tension, and the daily demands of diabetes may mean that life with diabetes is not always 'pleasurable'. Depression is prevalent among adults with diabetes (Lustman *et al.* 1992, Pita *et al.* 2002) and there is evidence that young people can also be psychologically affected (Kovacs *et al.* 1997a, 1997b).

Quality of life can be defined as how good or bad life is felt to be. This quality can be affected by both internal and external factors. These include an individual's personal characteristics, current health status, family circumstances, environment, concerns about the future, friendships and life at school or work. The quality of one's life as perceived by the individual is an important indicator of overall well-being and, for young people living with diabetes, may sometimes seem a more critical one than the quality of one's glycaemic control.

Individuals' quality of life, as well as their physiological health, is recognised as an outcome of diabetes management: if self management tasks become too onerous or relationships with health care staff are poor, for example, quality of life as well as bodily health can be affected. Despite the resilience of many of the young people who participated in the study, the comments of a minority show some of the negative effects of living with diabetes.

> I hate it. It's upsetting. I am worrying all the time. I worry
> about dying and being blind. I wish there was a cure.
> *(13 year old male)*

> There are times when I wish it would just go away if only for
> one day so I could forget about it because the fact that it is
> always there and won't go away is awful to live with.
> *(16 year old female)*

> With my diabetes I feel very uncomfortable because to
> myself I feel different to other people. I don't like this at all.
> *(13 year old female)*

However, studies have shown that good glycaemic control is associated with better quality of life and with better family relationships (Guttman-Bauman *et al.* 1998, Hoey *et al.* 2001). In response to this a number of diabetes services are offering psychological support to young people to help them take a more positive approach to living with the condition and, therefore, to help them enhance both glycaemic control and quality of life (Hampson *et al.* 2001). Support can be in the form of individual counselling or a course for a group of young people. This more holistic approach to diabetes management acknowledges that HbA1c levels are not the only product of treatment and that quality of life can also be used as a valid outcome measure (Eiser and Morse 2001).

In order to measure their perceived quality of life, young participants in the current study were asked to complete the ADDQoL-Teen questionnaire. The questionnaire was developed as a tool to measure both respondents' quality of life and the extent to which they believe that diabetes has an impact on that quality across a number of areas of their lives. The questionnaire was used to gain knowledge of how young people felt about their lives and how much they considered having diabetes positively or negatively affected it.

The quality of life questionnaire

As described in Chapter 4, the quality of life measure used in the study was developed specifically for young people aged 13 to 16 by psychologists at Royal Holloway, University of London. Qualitative work had earlier been carried out in four hospitals in Greater London (Wilson *et al.* 1998) and a literature review conducted. These identified important quality of life issues which formed the content of items included in the questionnaire. The items were designed to reflect young people's own perceptions of living with diabetes and to measure their feelings about the importance of the issues in their everyday lives. Young people's comments informed the development of questionnaire items, response choices and design. It is hoped that the ADDQoL-Teen will be used by health professionals to consider psychological issues as well as health outcomes when caring for young people with diabetes and that it will be useful in evaluating new treatments and educational interventions for diabetes in clinical trials.

The questionnaire opens with two overview items which are linked. The first is a statement about perceived quality of life in general and the second asks how much the respondent thinks having diabetes has an impact on quality of life. Like all the questions, each question has response boxes which the respondent is asked to mark. Quality of life is defined in the questionnaire as 'how good or bad you feel your life is'.

The two overview items and response boxes are:

1. In general, I feel my quality of life is

Brilliant	Good	OK	Not OK	Bad

2. Does diabetes usually make your quality of life worse or better?

A lot worse	A fair bit worse	A bit worse	Neither worse nor better	Better

The questionnaire goes on to cover 30 issues which were identified by young people in the development process as important to their lives with diabetes. Each question asks to what extent or how frequently an issue figures in respondents' lives and is followed by a linked question asking to what extent that issue has an impact. Each question has a series of response boxes. For example, Question 3 asks:

3a. Do you ever feel people fuss or worry about you because of your diabetes?

Yes – a lot	Yes – a fair bit	Yes – a bit	No – I do not

The following linked question asks:

3b. Does it bother you when people fuss or worry about you because of your diabetes?

Yes – it bothers me very much	Yes – it bothers me a fair bit	Yes – it bothers me a bit	No – it does not bother me, it's OK	No – it does not bother me, I like it

Other questions follow a similar format and all are followed by a subsequent question asking the respondent 'does it bother you when…?' A list of the questions included is shown below.

4. Do you ever feel you want to eat sweets but don't because of your diabetes?
5. Do you ever want to drink something but you don't drink it because of your diabetes?
6. Do you ever want to eat something but you don't eat it because of your diabetes?
7. Do you take insulin?
8. Do you ever bleed or have any bruises or lumpy bits where you take your insulin?
9. Do you ever have extra things, like snacks, money, treats or days out because of your diabetes?

10. Do you ever find diabetes interrupts what you are doing, like watching TV, working at home or school, playing computer games or any other activities?
11. Do you have finger prick blood tests?
12. Do you ever feel you want to take more control of diabetes on your own, with less help from other people?
13. Do changes in your blood sugars ever make you feel moody?
14. Do you ever feel unwell because of your diabetes, like having a headache or pain, or feeling tired, sick or dizzy?
15. Do you ever find that having diabetes gets you out of a fix, or gets you out of doing something you don't want to do?
16. Do you ever get asked to sleep away from home or at a friend's house, but you don't because of your diabetes?
17. Do you ever wake up in the night feeling hypo with low blood sugar?
18. Do you ever want to have a lie in bed, but don't because of your diabetes?
19. Do you ever miss a party, a school trip, going out or any other event because of your diabetes?
20. Do you ever feel your blood sugar is too low?
21. Do you ever feel your blood sugar is too high?
22. Do you ever worry about the future, like getting married, having children or your future health, because of your diabetes?
23. Do you ever feel that having diabetes will make a difference to your future job or career?
24. Do you ever feel 'different' because of your diabetes?
25. Are you ever told that things are 'not allowed' because of your diabetes?
26. Do you ever feel that diabetes makes a difference to life with your family or the people you live with?
27. Do you ever find you are expected to take more responsibility than you would like because of your diabetes?
28. Do you ever find that having diabetes makes any difference to playing sport?
29. Do you find that you need to go to the toilet too often because of your diabetes?
30. Do you ever find you need to fit diabetes into your social life, like carrying equipment, planning when to eat, or where to take insulin when away from home?
31. Do you go to a diabetes clinic?
32. Have you ever been on holidays or weekends away for young people with diabetes, or made new friends because of your diabetes?

The scores for the two parts of each question can then be multiplied to provide a weighted impact score for each issue or aspect of life. The majority of paired questions has negative sense but three ask about the potentially positive aspects of having diabetes – having extra treats, getting out of something unpleasant, and attending holidays or weekends away for young people with diabetes. These three are scored differently from the average weighted impact score. Two other items were not included in the average weighted impact score when the analysis was carried out. The first was 'do you ever get asked to sleep away from home or at a friend's house but you don't because of your diabetes?' to which almost 80 per cent responded 'No, I do not'. The second question was 'do you go to a diabetes clinic?' and was omitted from the weighted score because results of analysis of this item reduced the reliability of the whole scale.

There is space at the end of the questionnaire for individuals to make other comments about living with diabetes.

Results from the 'questionnaire sample'

Data from the 158 strong 'questionnaire sample' – those 78 young people who participated in the research study (i.e. the 78 of the 85 interviewed who completed a questionnaire) plus the 80 who filled in the questionnaire only – were used by psychologists at Royal Holloway to validate the quality of life measure. The data was tested for the homogeneity of the sample and for internal consistency and reliability and was found to be satisfactory. Completion rates for all questions were high, indicating the acceptability of the questionnaire to respondents. Although the questionnaire was developed for the 13 to 16 age group, it was expected that those aged 17 and 18 years could also complete it as many would be attending school or sixth form college. However, respondents in the sample were not all aged between 13 and 18. At the start of the project, the ages of young people attending adolescent and transition clinics were unknown and, in order to have comparable data, it was agreed to use the same questionnaire for all respondents. Over three-quarters (78 per cent) of the whole sample were attending school or sixth form college at the time of questionnaire completion. Table 10.1 shows the ages of the whole sample. More than 80 per cent were aged 13–18 years. There were 75 males (47 per cent) and 83 females (53 per cent) in the whole sample. For background information on the 'questionnaire sample', see Chapter 4.

Table 10.1 Ages of respondents in the 'questionnaire sample'

	n	%
10–12 years	7	4
13–16 years	99	63
17–18 years	31	20
19 years and over	21	13
Total	158	100

Results of the two overview items show that the majority of young people (71 per cent) felt that the quality of their lives was 'brilliant' or 'good' while nearly a quarter (24 per cent) thought it was 'OK' (Table 10.2). A small minority (7 individuals) felt life was 'not OK' or 'bad'.

Table 10.2 In general, I feel my quality of life is… ('questionnaire sample')

	n	%
Brilliant	27	17
Good	84	54
OK	37	24
Not OK	4	3
Bad	3	2
Total	155	100

Table 10.3 Does diabetes usually make your quality of life worse or better? ('questionnaire sample')

It makes it...	n	%
a lot worse	9	6
a fair bit worse	20	13
a bit worse	67	43
neither worse nor better	55	35
better	4	3
Total	155	100

Three respondents did not answer the above two questions

Over a third (35 per cent) felt that having diabetes made no difference to quality of life although 19 per cent thought having diabetes made life 'a fair bit worse' or 'a lot worse' (Table 10.3). Four young people thought having diabetes made their lives better. There was no statistically significant difference in response by age or sex of respondent. Comments added at the end of the questionnaires illustrate how many young people are pragmatic about living with diabetes.

> I don't like being diabetic but I haven't got much choice. It affects my life sometimes but most of the time I'm fine.
> *(15 year old male)*

> I've had diabetes since I was young so it makes no difference to my life at all because it's a routine I'm used to and everything just comes naturally.
> *(15 year old female)*

> As I've got older I've learned to accept being diabetic and I've learned being different isn't that horrible after all. Now I know doing blood tests and taking insulin is just part of my everyday routine. Diabetes is something that I've learned I've got to live with.
> *(16 year old female)*

> I am 17 years old and currently at college on a full-time course. My diabetes doesn't affect me in any way or stop me doing things. All my friends are aware of my condition and have no problems. I don't think it has affected my life a lot – simply made me more responsible.
> *(17 year old female)*

> When I first had diabetes, I felt like an outcast but now I accept it and most people, apart from some teachers, don't treat me different. Diabetes can even get me out of things like PE and housework!
> *(16 year old female)*

The areas of greatest importance to respondents in terms of frequency of the response 'Yes – a lot' were taking insulin (68 per cent), doing finger prick tests (47 per cent), fitting diabetes into social life (25 per cent) and wanting to eat sweets but not doing so because of diabetes (23 per cent). Three items were not experienced by the majority of respondents. These were missing a party, school trip or event because of diabetes (82 per cent), being asked to sleep away from home or at a friend's but not doing so because of diabetes (79 per cent), and going away for weekends or holidays for young people with diabetes or making new friends because of diabetes (72 per cent). These results show that respondents are most likely to experience the day to day routines of living with diabetes such as injecting insulin, blood testing and having to fit diabetes into social life (carrying equipment, planning where and when to eat and take insulin) and least likely to be prevented from participating in social events, including sleepovers, by having diabetes. Just over a quarter (27%) of respondents had been away on a weekend or holiday for young people with diabetes or made new friends through having diabetes.

The items in which the highest percentage of young people were very much bothered by having diabetes were feeling unwell because of diabetes (24 per cent), bleeding or having bruises or lumps at injection sites (21 per cent), having activities (both at school and in leisure time) interrupted (20 per cent) and feeling blood sugar is too high (20 per cent).

Respondents were asked if people fussed or worried about them and, although nearly all of them (97 per cent) answered that they did, over a quarter (28 per cent) were not bothered about being fussed over. Indeed five young people reported that they liked it. Similarly, all but one young person responded that they did finger prick blood tests but over half (53 per cent) did not mind doing them although 30 per cent said they were bothered 'very much' or 'a fair bit' by these tests.

One of the items included in the questionnaire was the frequency with which respondents attended a diabetes clinic and whether attendance bothered them. Results for these two items are shown in Tables 10.4 and 10.5. Three respondents reported that they did not attend a diabetes clinic (Table 10.4) and one failed to answer the question about whether they were bothered by attending (Table 10.5).

Table 10.4 Do you go to a diabetes clinic? ('questionnaire sample')

	n	%
Yes – a lot	36	23
Yes – a fair bit	85	54
Yes – a bit	34	21
No – I do not	3	2
Total	158	100

Table 10.5 Does going to the diabetes clinic bother you? ('questionnaire sample')

.	n	%
Yes – it bothers me very much	7	5
Yes – it bothers me a fair bit	10	6
Yes – it bothers me a bit	21	14
No – it doesn't bother me, it's OK	88	57
No – it doesn't bother me, I like it	28	18
Total	154	100

Over three-quarters (77 per cent) said they attended a diabetes clinic 'a lot' or 'a fair bit' and exactly three-quarters did not mind or liked going to the clinic. Of the quarter who were bothered by clinic visits, 14 per cent were bothered 'a bit' and 11 per cent 'very much' or 'a fair bit'. Evidence from the interviews with young people in the study showed that the majority were happy with the care they received from health services and results from this larger sample tally with those findings.

The items which resulted in the most severe negative impact of diabetes, in order of severity, were not being able to have a lie in, school work or leisure activities being interrupted, worrying about the future and eating sweets. The items that showed the least negative impact of diabetes, in order of least severity, were attending a diabetes clinic, having low blood sugar, being expected to take more responsibility, taking control of diabetes and waking up at night feeling hypo.

The 'interview sample'

Of the 85 young people who participated in the interviews, 78 completed the quality of life questionnaire at first interview. Their responses to the first two questions are shown in Tables 10.6 and 10.7.

Table 10.6 In general, I feel my quality of life is... ('interview sample')

	n	%
Brilliant	17	22
Good	45	58
OK	14	18
Not OK	1	1
Bad	1	1
Total	78	100

Table 10.7 Does diabetes usually make your quality of life worse or better? ('interview sample')

.	n	%
A lot worse	3	4
A fair bit worse	7	9
A bit worse	28	36
Neither worse nor better	37	47
Better	3	4
Total	78	100

The results show that those young people who participated in interviews were more likely to describe their quality of life as 'brilliant' or 'good' than those young people in the larger sample (80 per cent compared to 71 per cent) and less likely to describe it as 'not OK' or 'bad' (2 per cent compared to 5 per cent). The proportion of respondents aged over 16 was larger in this sample than in the whole sample and this accounts for the difference in results as the older respondents were more likely to report their quality of life as 'brilliant' or 'good' than the 13 to 16 year olds. Similarly the sample who were interviewed were more likely to believe that diabetes made their quality of life 'neither worse nor better' than the whole sample (47 per cent compared to 35 per cent) and less likely to report that diabetes made quality of life 'a lot' or 'a fair bit' worse (13 per cent compared to 19 per cent).

Analysis of the questionnaire data shows that on the whole respondents felt happy about their quality of life and, in their view, diabetes did not affect it greatly. However, a minority felt that their quality of life is no better than 'OK' and that diabetes has a severely negative impact. As guidelines for the care of young people with diabetes recommend that psychological support should be made available to them (British Diabetic Association 1995), a quality of life questionnaire aimed specifically at this age group is a useful assessment tool for practitioners as well as researchers.

11. Understanding diabetes: the information needs of young people

The person with diabetes is responsible for his or her own care on a daily basis and so needs to have enough information about and understanding of the condition to manage the everyday tasks of administering insulin and testing blood. Without the information they need to make judgements about their own care, young people with diabetes would be completely dependent on health care professionals and parents. It is recognised that a 'fundamental prerequisite for diabetes self-management is patient education' (Anderson *et al.* 1995) and the availability of accessible, up to date information is therefore an essential component of diabetes care. This chapter and the following one examine what hospital staff and young people said about diabetes education and information, the role of group activities and ideas for new information resources.

Patient empowerment

There are, of course, different sources of information available and also different types of knowledge. Traditionally, diabetes education has aimed to ensure that people with diabetes know enough to adhere to the treatment recommended by health care professionals. In recent years, however, the concept of 'patient empowerment' has transformed ideas about how best to educate people with a chronic condition. 'Patient empowerment' seeks to make people with diabetes experts in managing their condition and to teach them the necessary skills to allow them to make informed choices about their lives. This model recognises that 'human beings have physical, intellectual, emotional, social and spiritual components to their lives that interact in a holistic and dynamic fashion' (Feste 1992) and that they have both the right and the responsibility to make decisions that concern them. The patient is seen as the primary manager of chronic disease while health care professionals act to guide and educate (Clark and Gong 2000).

Staff members who were interviewed for the study described how they try to both provide diabetes education to young people and encourage them to use their knowledge to make well informed decisions about their care. Their view is that the more young people know and the more skilled they become in self-care then the more opportunity they will have to follow a lifestyle that suits them while maintaining good glycaemic control.

> We try and empower them absolutely so they can do a lot of
> it themselves. They have written material, they have teaching
> dedicated to adjusting insulin, they have videos, they have
> access to all of that information on the web.
> *(Consultant paediatrician)*

Sources of information

Information about diabetes is provided by means of books, leaflets and booklets, magazines, CD-Roms, videos and websites. These are produced by a wide range of organisations including Diabetes UK, pharmaceutical companies and hospital services. Two of the services included in the study have their own web pages which include information about the service. One site offers advice on diet, hypoglycaemia, travel and adjusting insulin dose. At another hospital, the diabetes specialist nurse provides a noticeboard for the adolescent clinic where she pins up to date information about all aspects of diabetes and diabetes care including items on genetic research and newly available products. This acts both to inform young people as they wait to see the doctor and as a talking point to encourage discussion. Short pieces of information which are to the point and do not take long to read are popular.

> Leaflets that you could pick up and take away. Maybe not have
> one big one, but have separate little ones on all the different
> aspects of it so you could just take what interests you.
> *(19 year old female)*

Perhaps the most important source of information, however, is provided during face to face, individualised discussions between staff members and young people and their families which occur in the clinic, on the telephone or at home. If sufficient time is available, these are interactive sessions when young people (and perhaps their parents) have the opportunity to ask questions and return to particular issues they want clarified. As noted in Chapter 3, motivated young people in research area E have been given the opportunity to learn more about diabetes. It is hoped that their enhanced knowledge will enable them to improve their glycaemic control more independently.

All services in the study have experimented with group activities and young people are also able to attend family weekends or activity holidays organised by Diabetes UK or by the diabetes service.

Reinforcing education

Clearly information about diabetes should be available at the appropriate time and level for young people to be able to make best use of it and 'individual treatment goals should take into account the patient's capacity to understand and carry out the treatment regimen' (American Diabetes Association 1994). One concern has been that young people who are diagnosed as babies or small children may need to be re-educated as adolescents because they may actually understand little about diabetes despite having lived with it for many years. Education is directed towards parents if the child is very young at diagnosis and although parents may think they have passed on their knowledge it may not have necessarily transferred to the child. One study found, for example, that young people who were unable to explain the nature of diabetes were likely to have been diagnosed at an early age (Challen *et al.* 1993).

A nurse and a young woman who were interviewed acknowledged this problem.

> You have to be careful because what happens is for years parents have always done it and they actually think they're teaching their children about it but actually they're keeping some of it to themselves ... They do it automatically, so sometimes they don't give all the information to the child and expect them to be able to do everything.
> *(Paediatric diabetes specialist nurse)*

> I think I've forgotten quite a lot – things I got taught when I was nine.
> *(18 year old female)*

This suggests that diabetes education should be ongoing: as young people mature they understand more and as they grow more independent are increasingly able to put that understanding into practice in their daily lives.

Transfer to adult care can be an opportunity for staff in the adult service to reinforce some of the education young people have already received from parents and paediatric staff. They may take a different approach to that of their paediatric colleagues which may interest or engage the young person anew. Health care staff must also ensure that young people are kept informed about new developments and treatments in diabetes. Without knowledge about the availability of particular devices, young people would not be in a position to take an active part in decision making about their care.

What the young people said

During interviews young people were asked whether they felt they had enough information about diabetes and where they would look for information if they felt they needed it. The large majority of young people (86 per cent) said that they felt they had enough information to care for themselves. When asked where they would seek additional information, 90 per cent said they would ask the diabetes specialist nurse at their next clinic appointment and, if it was urgent, they would telephone the nurse. Others would talk to one of their parents, particularly if that parent also had diabetes, or the doctor. Three said they had used the internet for information about diabetes and another had learned a lot working at a camp for children with diabetes in the United States. One 20 year old said that having access to the internet at university had taught him more about diabetes than he had learned since he was diagnosed at the age of 12.

However, young people who participated in the study were not tested on their knowledge of diabetes and it may be that, for some, it was limited. One, for example, said, 'I think I know enough but not everything that I need' (15 year old male) and another admitted to not wanting to 'look in an encyclopaedia and read up about it' (17 year old male). Two complained that they were told the same things over and over again at clinic appointments which they felt was counter-productive to learning.

Information in the form of leaflets that could be taken away from the clinic was valued, particularly that related to the effects of smoking, drinking and taking drugs on diabetes. The mother of one 16 year old male felt that not enough information was available for adolescents about the medical complications of diabetes.

> I don't think there's enough information for youngsters
> to tell them the side-effects of mismanaging your diabetes.
> I don't think children know that soon enough. They ain't
> even talked to us about alcohol in your sleep or smoking
> or anything else.

The question of when and how to raise these kinds of subjects is not simple. As discussed above, young people may feel they are facing an inquisition when asked by health care staff about their 'risk-taking behaviour' and those still at school are no doubt also being counselled about the hazards of smoking, drugs, alcohol and having sex by teaching staff. It is vital, however, that young people with diabetes are informed about the risks to their health of, for example, smoking or drinking alcohol, but it should be done in such a way that does not frighten them into a state of denial. One young woman admitted that she was afraid to know too much about diabetes.

> I think to a certain extent I choose not to look at it in
> too much detail because it scares me really. I do get very
> concerned about my long-term health and that's caused
> quite a lot of anxiety for me recently. Things like my
> eyesight and having children and things like that.
> *(18 year old female)*

Young people were also asked about whether hospital staff had discussed diet and body weight, exercise, smoking, drinking alcohol, drug use and sex and relationships with them. Of those young people who had not yet transferred to adult care, just over half (52 per cent) had discussed diet and exercise with a doctor but fewer than half said they had discussed the other issues. Doctors were least likely to have talked about drugs (29 per cent) or sex and relationships (24 per cent) (Table 11.1). Similarly a majority of young people reported that they had not talked to a nurse about any of these issues although half had discussed drinking alcohol with a nurse and were more likely to have talked about sex and relationships with a nurse than a doctor (38 per cent) (Table 11.2). Over half (55 per cent) of those who had not yet transferred to adult care had talked to a dietician about diet but 65 per cent had not discussed exercise.

Table 11.1 Have you talked to the doctor about lifestyle?

	Diet and body weight		Exercise		Alcohol		Drugs		Smoking		Sex and relationships	
	n	%	n	%	n	%	n	%	n	%	n	%
Before transfer												
Yes	22	52	22	52	20	48	12	29	17	40	10	24
No	20	48	20	48	22	52	30	71	25	60	31	74
Not sure											1	2
After transfer												
Yes	19	44	20	47	13	30	4	9	11	26	4	9
No	23	54	22	51	28	65	39	91	32	74	37	86
Not sure	1	2	1	2	2	5					2	5

Table 11.2 Have you talked to the nurse about lifestyle?

	Diet and body weight		Exercise		Alcohol		Drugs		Smoking		Sex and relationships	
	n	%	n	%	n	%	n	%	n	%	n	%
Before transfer												
Yes	18	43	18	43	21	50	11	26	16	38	16	38
No	23	55	23	55	21	50	30	72	25	60	25	60
Not sure	1	2	1	2			1	2	1	2	1	2
After transfer												
Yes	12	28	13	30	13	30	7	16	9	21	7	16
No	29	67	28	65	28	65	34	79	32	74	34	79
Not sure	2	5	2	5	2	5	2	5	2	5	2	5

The majority who had transferred to adult care said they had not talked about
these issues to either a doctor or a nurse. This may be because they had recently
transferred and had only attended one or two appointments at the adult clinic.
These results are worrying. Although staff reported that discussion of these
issues is a necessary part of diabetes education for young people, many young
people deny having talked to staff about them. In some cases, they may have
forgotten the discussion or been too embarrassed to mention it but it seems
important that staff ensure that these issues are raised at clinic appointments
(or at other times) and that young people are given the information they need.

Young people were also asked if they or their families received magazines produced by Diabetes UK. More than half (52 per cent) did receive them although eight said that they used to get them but did not any longer and had not considered why not (Table 11.3). Presumably membership of Diabetes UK had lapsed. Of the 44 who received magazines, 15 said they read them regularly, 23 read them occasionally and the other six did not read them although their parents did.

Table 11.3 Do you see Diabetes UK magazines?

.	n	%
Yes	44	52
No	30	35
Used to	8	10
Don't know	3	3
Total	85	100

Learning together – group activities

Although staff at all clinics reported having experimented with organising group activities either during clinics or at other times, these had had limited success in terms of their attractiveness to young people. Some initiatives, such as holidays for children with diabetes, are popular but others, educational sessions during clinics, for example, have not met with approval as young people have made it clear that they do not feel comfortable about shared activities. Young people were asked if there were such activities at their clinic and, if so, whether they had participated in them. Interestingly, although over a quarter (26 per cent) reported that there were group activities, more than 60 per cent said they did not know if group activities were organised or not (Table 11.4).

Table 11.4 Does the clinic organise educational sessions or group discussions?

.	n	%
Yes	22	26
No	11	13
Not sure	52	61
Total	85	100

Of the 22 who said that the clinic did organise group activities, only five said they had attended one. However, despite the mixed reaction to such activities reported by members of staff, over half (56 per cent) of those interviewed said they would be interested in meeting other young people with diabetes although 39 per cent qualified this by responding that they would 'maybe' like to meet others (Table 11.5). More than half (57 per cent) said they knew at least one person with diabetes in their own age group.

Table 11.5 Would you like to meet other people with diabetes?

.	n	%
Yes, definitely	15	17
Yes, maybe	33	39
No	37	44
Total	85	100

How such meetings could be arranged and in what location is something diabetes team members might consider, although the experiences described by staff members show that young people may say they are interested in particular activities but may not turn up when they are arranged. As noted above, staff at all clinics had tried to stimulate group outings, discussions or education sessions but found that these were time consuming (and sometimes expensive) to organise and that it was difficult to sustain interest. At one hospital, for example, a group of young people had met away from the clinic and made a video about having diabetes. This activity was a great success but staff found it could not be repeated the following year as the cohort of young people did not seem willing to work together in the same way and it was hard for staff to maintain the momentum and resources to facilitate further out of clinic activities. These experiences illustrate how difficult it is for staff who are already working at full capacity to organise events and activities and how their enthusiasm can be dulled by young people for whom diabetes related activities may be seen as 'uncool'.

Other examples of group activities are sessions where young people can discuss techniques and approaches which help them cope with living with diabetes. One of the hospitals involved in the study was running a research project and one aspect of this was to offer group sessions to young people with the aim of developing a protocol for such groups which could be made available to other diabetes services. The sessions were facilitated by two psychologists who were encouraging participants to take a solution focused approach to their lives, concentrating on themselves as people rather than on diabetes as a problem. Although only a minority of young people using the diabetes service had chosen to join the groups, few dropped out during the six week course. The sessions were held in the hospital after school hours which may have posed problems for those who did not live nearby.

Young people were asked if they had attended camps run by Diabetes UK or their local diabetes service (see Table 11.6). These holidays provide children and young people with a valuable opportunity to learn by experience in a context that is very different from the hospital clinic. Holidays can include activities such as abseiling or caving and young people have to learn to adjust their food intake, level of exercise and insulin dose to deal with unfamiliar and strenuous exercise. They also offer young people a chance to meet others with diabetes socially. These holidays are staffed by health professionals who act as volunteers. Forty-three (27 per cent) of the 'questionnaire sample' had attended at least one holiday and of these over half (56 per cent) said they liked it 'a fair bit' or 'a lot'. Some of those who were interviewed reported that they had attended a camp or weekend away when they were younger.

Table 11.6 Have you ever been on a camp for children or young people with diabetes?

	n	%
More than once	15	18
Once	10	12
Never	60	70
Total	85	100

One 23 year old man had attended Diabetes UK's youth weekends which he found useful in terms of learning about diabetes. Although the weekends are attended by health care professionals, he found it particularly rewarding to talk to other people like himself – who were young and had diabetes.

> I've been surrounded by 70 or 80 other diabetics plus medical staff there who specialise in diabetes. That has probably been the biggest source of information that I've had ... Just talking to people who are in a similar situation, who have had similar problems ... because you can talk to health care professionals or whatever, but if they haven't got it themselves, it's often very difficult for them. They could

> have all the information in the world but until you've been
> hypo or hyper, you often don't realise quite what it's like, so
> just talking to those other people who are in the same
> situation, the same age group, the same problems or
> whatever and also talking to people who really specialise in
> diabetes care was a great help.

Others were definite that they did not want to be defined by having diabetes and
would rather not be involved with other people with diabetes for that reason.

> It's always been with me if there was a train with diabetic
> people and a train with non-diabetic people – it's not that
> I'm ashamed or anything of being diabetic – I'd get on the
> second one. It sounds bad but I don't really think that I've
> got it really, you know.
> *(18 year old female)*

Diabetes education is a vital part of diabetes care for all age groups. It is
particularly important for young people at the time when they are developing
greater understanding and leading increasingly independent lives. Information
can be made available through written materials and other media including
videos, CD-Roms and the internet and, perhaps most importantly, during
conversations with health care staff. Staff should ensure that they raise
appropriate topics with young people, particularly those that relate to behaviour
that may be risky for their health in both the short and long term. All young
people need to know about the effects of alcohol on blood glucose levels, for
example, and young women should be counselled about pregnancy and diabetes.

12. Diabetes and the internet

An aim of this study was to explore the availability of information resources for young people with diabetes. Although there is a wide range of written material available for children and young people (and their families) as well as CD-Roms and videos, there is a gap in information provided for this age group on the internet. There are some relevant websites but there are currently very few interactive online resources dedicated to young people with diabetes.

In order to find out how likely it would be that young people would make use of such a site, respondents were asked if they had access to the internet and, if they did, where. The large majority (86 per cent) said they had internet access, either at home (57 per cent) or at school, college or work (63 per cent). Others had access at a library or at a friend's home. Almost all of those interviewed said they would find information about diabetes on the internet useful. However, only a fifth of those who had access said they had looked at diabetes related websites. Many were attracted by the idea of a diabetes related chat-room or message board where individuals' experiences could be shared anonymously. Over half (59 per cent) of the young people with internet access had used chat-rooms.

Consulting young people about their information needs

In order to investigate what kinds of information young people want access to and what formats they find attractive, researchers organised a Diabetes Internet Day. The aim was to consult young people about their information needs, find out what they thought of existing diabetes related websites and generate ideas about what a website for young people might include and how it might look.

Leaflets promoting the day were sent to diabetes specialist nurses in the London area to display in clinics and hand out to young people attending appointments. Four young people from Edinburgh who had worked together on a health promotion leaflet were also invited and travelled to London with their diabetes specialist nurse. Fourteen young people aged between 13 and 18 attended in all, plus researchers and representatives from Diabetes UK.

Sessions on the day focused on information needs and how these might be met by an internet site, an evaluation of existing diabetes related websites, anonymity and security of chat-rooms and the components of an ideal internet site for young people with diabetes.

Existing online information for young people with diabetes

Staff in the Library and Information Service at the National Children's Bureau carried out an audit of existing websites. There are excellent health related sites for young people but these have limited information about diabetes. Although there is an American site specifically aimed at children with diabetes, only one UK site was found. Diabetes Explained (www.diabetes-explained.co.uk) was set up by Dominic Patterson, one of the research project's advisory group members. The site includes information about how diabetes affects the body, as well as links to other sites and a message board that can be used by visitors to the site. There is a small group of young people who are in regular e-mail contact via this site and the message board seems to play a supportive role for those who use it.

What young people want from a website

Young people who attended the Diabetes Internet Day were asked to think about an ideal website that would be both attractive to users and provide the kind of information they want to access.

General principles

Participants felt it was important that a website should have input from young people with diabetes themselves because 'kids know what kids like' and 'adults could get it checked by kids'. Information should be produced in short, accessible chunks with the facility for finding out more detail by clicking. The site should be attractive and fun to use. It could be used as a leisure activity and not a task. Cartoons and cartoon characters could be used, particularly to attract younger children.

Features

Some ideas for features:

- Diary of a person with diabetes
- The thoughts and experiences of famous people who have diabetes
- A website based on a character or characters (see, for example, www.teenagehealthfreak.com)
- A page for people who do not have diabetes to explain it in an interesting way which could include how a friend can help if you have a hypo
- animated games (relevant to diabetes)

Treating diabetes

Advice on:

- symptoms and diagnosis
- dealing with hypos/hypers
- 'just in case' – carry a kit with you, have some money for food, take extra insulin
- complications of diabetes
- injection sites
- insulin and how it works

Food and drink

- 'nice', easy to make recipes
- how to eat badly and get away with it!
- ideas for how to approach schools about improving school dinners
- how to check ingredients of foods and drinks
- how to drink alcohol safely
- managing weight

Feelings

How to deal with feeling:

- uncomfortable in social situations
- angry
- jealous
- upset
- scared

Relationships

- living with other family members
- telling friends and boy/girlfriends about diabetes
- how to respond to people who may be ignorant about diabetes
- how to deal with negative reactions from others
- making the best of consultations with doctors and nurses

Dissemination

- information on diabetes related events including holidays for children and young people with diabetes

School and college

- dealing with bullying
- getting support from teachers and friends
- information for teachers and other school staff about diabetes
- sport and diabetes
- school trips and diabetes
- exams and diabetes

Growing up

- general advice on alcohol and drug use
- leaving home and how to access medical care away from home (especially at university)

- eating new types of food and cooking for yourself
- changes of routine and lifestyle
- sex, relationships, contraception, pregnancy
- legal implications of having diabetes in relation to careers and leisure activities

Travelling abroad

- what to take and how to carry insulin, etc.
- types of insulin available in different countries
- how to access medical help abroad
- telling new friends about diabetes
- diabetes and activities (white water rafting, trekking, climbing, sailing)

Research and development in diabetes management

- young people's reviews of new products (pens, meters, etc.)
- readable research reports, e.g. genetic research, new methods taking insulin

Interaction

- chat-room/message board to communicate and share experiences with other young people who are living with diabetes
- online consultation with a doctor or nurse
- quizzes testing what you know about diabetes
- competitions

Links

- a page of hyperlinks to other relevant sites (not necessarily only diabetes related)

A large proportion of young people have access to the internet and young people with diabetes could use this medium for information and to make contact with others in similar circumstances for support and advice. A website dedicated to young people with diabetes, which was backed by sufficient resources to allow it to be regularly updated and to offer opportunities for interaction, would be well received by this group and would allow them to choose the level of information they wanted to make use of. The increase in young people continuing their education beyond the age of 16 means that there is a growing number who use computers and the internet routinely and with confidence. A website that was well designed, accurate and provided up to date information would be a valuable resource for this group of young people. Young people themselves should be able to participate in its development.

13. Conclusion

This report is based on the views of young people with diabetes on diabetes
services, the transition to adult care, their relationships with family and friends,
their experiences at school and college and their feelings about the quality of
their lives. The opinions and aspirations of health care staff who work with these
young people have also been included. This concluding chapter aims to provide
a brief overview of the issues discussed in the report with recommendations
about how services could improve to meet the needs of this special group of
young people, particularly in relation to the transfer of their care from
paediatric to adult services.

Young people with diabetes

Young people with diabetes are a heterogeneous group living in different
circumstances and having different needs. Some may have had diabetes for as
long as they can remember while others have been recently diagnosed. Some
have a family member or members who also have diabetes and some are the
only person they know who has it. Their responses to the challenges of
managing diabetes will also be different and are determined by variables such as
age, social and family circumstances and personality. A number of respondents
wrote their thoughts about having diabetes on the last page of the quality of life
questionnaire. Some described their frustration with the condition while others
had a more positive attitude.

> I feel it has to be one of the worst things that has happened
> to me in my whole life.
> *(15 year old female)*

I don't think it has affected my life a lot – simply made me
more responsible.
(17 year old female)

Why me??? Why me???
(13 year old male)

Diabetes can even get me out of things like PE and
housework!
(16 year old female)

Despite their differences, however, and like adults with diabetes, the health
outcomes of these young people will be affected by determinants such as socio-
economic status, ethnicity and lifestyle. Unlike their peers at school and college,
they will all be in the process of taking on the responsibilities of diabetes
management as they grow to adulthood. This means handling the daily
interactions of eating, taking insulin and exercising while also coping with the
new demands of emerging independence. These young people will be forging
new identities, forming new relationships and perhaps experimenting with
alcohol and drugs as well as facing changes in their diabetes care and, possibly,
discrimination at school or work. If their glycaemic control is poor during
adolescence, they will live in the shadow of the diabetes related complications
that they may have to confront in adulthood.

Data from the interviews with young people and from the questionnaires show
that most young people in the sample are positive about their quality of life, are
socially and psychologically well adjusted, attend most of their clinic
appointments and are generally happy with the care that they receive. Despite
their resilience to change, there is evidence that some young people do find it
difficult to manage diabetes in the adolescent years and may need access to
psychological support. Although the majority are likely to do well, having
diabetes is a risk factor for psychological disorders (Grey *et al.* 1998) and girls
worry more than boys about diabetes and therefore could be more likely to
suffer from depression. The Audit Commission (2000) reported that 'few
hospitals had dedicated psychological support for people with diabetes' and the
current study found that in only one of six research sites were psychologists
included as an integral part of the multidisciplinary team. There is evidence
that psychological problems can influence adherence to treatment (Turner and
Kelly 2000) and it would therefore enhance services for young people with
diabetes if psychological support was easily accessible.

As discussed in Chapter 4, the sample of young people who participated in the study did not include a cohort of non-attenders of diabetes clinics and therefore the views and experiences of this group are not included. However, diabetes specialist nurses at the research hospitals actively encouraged young people to remain in contact with diabetes services and chased up those who defaulted. There should be mechanisms in place to keep in touch with young people who fail to attend clinic appointments. These need to be particularly foolproof at the point of transfer to adult care.

Relationships with staff

Interviews with staff members illustrate the potential difficulties of caring for adolescents who may be unwilling to communicate. Despite the balancing act staff described of encouraging young people without threatening them, the majority had succeeded in establishing a rapport. This was particularly true of diabetes specialist nurses who were popular with young patients and who were able to meet with them at home or between clinic appointments. However, a minority of young people thought doctors did not treat them with understanding or respect and some found doctors patronising. Young people liked members of staff who seemed to understand their lifestyles and who were not judgemental. It was suggested by one paediatric nurse that training in working with adolescents would be useful.

Transition to adult care

Research has shown that there is variation in the quality of diabetes care for adults, children and adolescents (Audit Commission 2000, Jefferson *et al.* 2003). Despite the efforts of health care staff to provide appropriate care for young people as they move to adult care, data from this study shows that many young people may not be very well prepared for the transition to adult care. Although the majority said that they felt ready to move up when the time came, many were vague about the transition process because they said they had not been consulted or given the opportunity to discuss it.

Standard 6 of the National Service Framework on Diabetes (DH 2001) states that all young people will experience a 'smooth transition' of care from paediatric to adult services. The Scottish Diabetes Framework asserts that 'children and young people should be treated in environments appropriate for their age group' (Scottish Executive 2001). To be 'smooth' the transition should be clearly defined but also flexible. It should fit into a service that is comprehensive, integrated and responsive to the needs of children, young people and adults with diabetes.

Staff who were interviewed for the study were in the process, where possible, of developing appropriate services for adolescents and young adults but could take a more standardised approach to explaining the process of moving to adult care to their patients *before* they were actually referred on. Information, including written information in the form of a letter or leaflet, should be made available and each young person's unique circumstances taken into account when preparing them for transfer. They should be allowed to participate in decision making about their care and given the opportunity to voice their concerns about transfer. Structures that allow them to meet at least once with adult staff before they move up would be reassuring for those who lack confidence about the move. If there is no young adult clinic in place, these young people are likely to experience busier clinics with a smaller ratio of staff to patients when they graduate to adult services. This is also the point at which they are more likely to default from clinic attendance completely.

Outside the clinic

Although the study focused on clinic arrangements for young people, the importance of family and peer relationships was also highlighted by participants. Home visits by diabetes specialist nurses were valued by young people, giving them a chance to consult with a professional in an informal, familiar setting. These home visits also offered nursing staff insights into individual young people's circumstances which were valuable in helping them to manage diabetes. Visits to schools by specialist nurses give teachers and other school staff the opportunity to learn about diabetes. Teachers are keen to learn and have expressed 'great relief' when the 'mystique' of diabetes has been removed (Carson 1998). The role of a diabetes specialist nurse dedicated to working with teenagers and young adults could provide the extra resource needed to ensure that young people can be seen outside the clinic setting. Such a role could also be used to follow up young people who have failed to attend clinic appointments.

Supporting young people's self-care

Young people cannot be empowered to take control of their own condition if they are not well informed and educated at a level that is appropriate for them as individuals. Information should be available through all media, including the internet, and education should be a continuous and interactive process. New products and treatments, such as the DAFNE (dose adjustment for normal eating) programme (DAFNE Study Group 2002), should be made available and young people be given choices about treatment regimens in order to ensure that they are recognised as central members of the care team.

References

Acerini, C L, Cheetham, T D, Edge, J A and Dunger, D B (2000) Both insulin sensitivity and insulin clearance in children and young adults with type 1 (insulin dependent) diabetes vary with growth hormone concentrations and with age, *Diabetologia*, 43, 1, 61-8

Akerblom, H K, Vaarala, O, Hyoty, H, Ilonen, J and Knip, M (2002) Environmental factors in the aetiology of type 1 diabetes, *American Journal of Medical Genetics*, 115, 1, 18-29

Allen, C, Zaccaro, D J, Palta, M, Klein, R, Duck, S C and d'Alessio, D J (1992) Glycaemic control in early IDDM. The Wisconsin Diabetes Registry, *Diabetes Care*, 15, 8, 980-7

American Diabetes Association (1994) Standards of medical care for patients with diabetes mellitus, *Diabetes Care*, 17, 6, 616-23

Anderson, R M, Funnell, M M, Butler, P M, Arnold, M S, Fitzgerald, J T and Feste, C C (1995) Patient empowerment, *Diabetes Care*, 18, 7, 943-9

Audit Commission (2000) *Testing times: a review of diabetes services in England and Wales*. Audit Commission

Bateman, J (1990) An extra source of conflict? Diabetes in adolescence, *Professional Nurse*, March, 290-6

Betts, P R, and Swift, P G F (2003) Doctor, who will be looking after my child's diabetes?, *Archives of Disease in Childhood*, 88, 6-7

Betts, P R, Jefferson, I G and Swift, P G F (2002) Diabetes care in childhood and adolescence, *Diabetes Medicine*, 19, Supplement 4, July, 61-5

Blum, R W, Garell, D, Hodgman, C H, Jorissen, T W, Okinow, N A, Orr, D P and Slap, G B, (1993) Transition from child-centred to adult health care for adolescents with chronic conditions. A position paper of the Society for Adolescent Medicine, *Journal of Adolescence Health*, 14, 7, 570-6

Bolton, A (1997) *Losing the thread: pupils' and parents' voices about education for sick children*. National Association for the Education of Sick Children

Branson, J and Ellerby, S (1997) Sweet and sour, *Health Service Journal*, 27 March, 37

Brink, S J (1997) So what's the difference between teenage boys and girls, anyway?, *Diabetes Care,* 20, 11, 1638-9

British Diabetic Association (BDA) (1995) *The principles of good practice for the care of young people with diabetes.* BDA

Bruining, G J for the Netherlands Kolibrie study group of childhood diabetes (2000) Association between infant growth before the onset of juvenile type 1 diabetes and autoantibodies to 1A-2, *The Lancet,* 365, 9230, 655-56

Bryden, K S, Neil, A, Mayou, R A, Peveler, R C, Fairburn, C G and Dunger, D B (1999) Eating habits, body weight, and insulin misuse. A longitudinal study of teenagers and young adults with type 1 diabetes, *Diabetes Care,* 22, 12

Bryden, K S, Peveler, R, Stein, A, Neil, A, Mayou, R A and Dunger, D B (2001) Clinical and psychological course of diabetes from adolescence to young adulthood: a longitudinal cohort study, *Diabetes Care,* 24, 9, 1513-14

Burden, M L, Burden, A C and Butterworth, S (1990) Diabetes education and schools, *Practical Diabetes,* 7, 5, 211-14

Carson, C (1998) Innovative approach to improving care for diabetic adolescents, *Journal of Diabetes Nursing,* 2, 4, 108-11

Carson, C (2000) A diabetic service for adolescents, *Nursing Times,* 96, 4, 43-4

Carson, C A and Kelnar, C J H (2000) The adolescent with diabetes, *Journal of the Royal College of Physicians of London,* 34, 1, 24-7

Challen, A H, Davies, A G, Baum, J D and Williams, R J W (1993) Adolescents' views about glycaemic control, *Practical Diabetes,* 10, 1, 26-30

Clark, N M and Gong, M (2000) Management of chronic disease by practitioners and patients: are we teaching the wrong things?, *British Medical Journal,* 320, 573-5

Coulter, A (2002) Patients' views of the good doctor, *British Medical Journal,* 325, 668-9

Cradock, S (1998) Managing to empower?, *Nursing Times,* 94, 35, 69-71

DAFNE Study Group (2002) Training in flexible, intensive insulin management to enable dietary freedom in people with type 1 diabetes: dose adjustment for normal eating (DAFNE) randomized control trial, *British Medical Journal,* 325, 746

David, T J (2001) Transition from the paediatric clinic to the adult service, *Journal of the Royal Society of Medicine,* 94, 8, 373-4

Delamater, A M, Jacobson, A M, Anderson, B, Cox, D, Fisher, L, Lustman, P, Rubin, R. and Wysocki, T, Psychological Therapies Working Group (2001) Psychosocial therapies in diabetes: report of the Psychological Therapies Working Group, *Diabetes Care,* 24, 7, 1286-92

Department for Education and Employment (DfEE) (1996) *Supporting pupils with medical needs*. DfEE

Department of Health (DH) (2001) *National Service Framework for Diabetes: Standards.* Department of Health

Department of Health (DH) (2003) *National Service Framework for Diabetes: Delivery Strategy*. Department of Health

Diabetes Control and Complications Trial (DCCT) Research Group (1993) The effect of intensive treatment of diabetes on the development and progression of long term complications in insulin-dependent diabetes mellitus, *New England Journal of Medicine*, 329, 14, 977-86

Drake, A J, Smith, A, Betts, P R, Crowe, E C and Shield, J P H (2002) Type 2 diabetes in obese white children, *Archives of Disease in Childhood*, 86, 207-8

du Pasquier-Fediaevsky, L and Tubiana-Rufi N, the PEDIAB Collaborative Group (1999) Discordance between physician and adolescent assessments of adherence to treatment: influence of HbA1c level, *Diabetes Care*, 22, 9, 1445-9

Dyer, O (2002) First cases of type 2 diabetes found in white UK teenagers, *British Medical Journal*, 324, 506

Dyer, P H, Lloyd, C E, Lancashire, R J, Bain, S C and Barnett, A H (1998) Factors associated with clinic non-attendance in adults with type 1 diabetes mellitus, *Diabetes Medicine*, 15, 4, 339-43

Edge, J A, Ford-Adams, M E and Dunger, D B (1999) Causes of death in children with insulin dependent diabetes 1990-96, *Archives of Disease in Childhood*, 61, 318-23

Eiser, C 'Observations about outpatient's clinics, with special reference to diabetes' *in* Kurtz, Z and Hopkins, A (1996) *Services for young people with chronic disorders in their transition from childhood to adult life*. Royal College of Physicians

Eiser, C and Morse, R (2001) A review of measures of quality of life for children with chronic illness, *Archives of Disease in Childhood*, 84, 205-11

Feltbower, R G, McKinney, P A and Bodansky, H J (2000) Rising incidence of childhood diabetes is seen at all ages and in urban and rural settings in Yorkshire, United Kingdom, *Diabetologia*, 43, 5, 682-4

Feste, C (1992) A practical look at patient empowerment, *Diabetes Care*, 15, 7, 922-5

Follansbee, D S (1989) Assuming responsibility for diabetes management: What age? What price?, *The Diabetes Educator*, 15, 347-51

Gale, E A and Gillespie, K M (2001) Diabetes and gender, *Diabetologia*, 44, 3-15

Gardner, S G, Bingley, P J, Sawtell, P A, Weeks, S and Gale, E A M, the Bart's-Oxford Study Group (1997) Rising incidence of insulin dependent diabetes in children aged under 5 years in the Oxford region: time trend analysis, *British Medical Journal*, 315, 713-17

Gill, G (1993) Diabetes in teenagers, *Maternal and Child Health*, August, 243-4

Green, A, Gale, E A M and Patterson, C C for the EURODIAB ACE Study Group (1992) Incidence of childhood-onset insulin-dependent diabetes mellitus: the EURODIAB ACE study, *The Lancet,* 339, April, 905-9

Grey, M, Boland, E A, Yu, C, Sullivan-Bolyai, S and Tamborlane, W V (1998) Personal and family factors associated with quality of life in adolescents with diabetes, *Diabetes Care*, 21, 6, 909-14

Griffin, S. (1998) Diabetes care in general practice: a meta-analysis of randomised control trials, *British Medical Journal*, 317, 390-4

Guttmann-Bauman, J, Flaherty, A P, Strugger, M and McEvoy, R C (1998) Metabolic control and quality of life self-assessment in adolescents with IDDM, *Diabetes Care*, 21, 6, 915-18

Hampson, S E, Skinner, T C, Hart, J, Storey, L, Gage, H, Foxcroft, D, Kimber, A, Shaw, K and Walker, J (2001) Effects of educational and psychosocial interventions for adolescents with diabetes mellitus: a systematic review, *Health Technology Assessment*, 5, 10

Hanson, C L, Hengeller, S W and Burghen, G A (1987) Social competence and parental support as mediators of the link between stress and metabolic control in adolescents with IDDM, *Journal of Consulting and Clinic Psychology*, 55, 4, 529-33

Hardy, K J, O'Brien, S V and Furlong, N J (2002) Information given to patients before appointments and its effect on non-attendance rate, *British Medical Journal*, 323, 1298-1300

Hoey, H, Aanstoot, H-J, Chiarelli, F, Daneman, D, Danne, T, Dorchy, H, Fitzgerald, M, Garandeau, P, Greene, S, Holl, R, Hougaard, P, Kaprio, E, Kocova, M, Lynggaard, H, Martul, P, Matsuura, N, McGee, H M, Mortensen, H B, Robertson, K, Schoenle, E, Sovik, O, Swift, P, Tsou, R M, Vanelli, M and Åman, J for the Hvidøre Study Group on Childhood Diabetes (2001) Good metabolic control is associated with better quality of life in 2101 adolescents with type 1 diabetes, *Diabetes Care*, 24, 11, 1923-8

Holman, H, and Lorig, K (2000) Patients as partners in managing chronic disease, *British Medical Journal*, 320, 526-7

ISPAD (2000) *Consensus Guidelines 2000: ISPAD consensus guidelines for the management of type 1 diabetes mellitus in children and adolescents.* International Society for Paediatric and Adolescent Diabetes

Jefferson, I G, Swift, P G F, Skinner, T C and Hood, G (2003) Diabetes services in the UK: third national survey confirms continuing deficiencies, *Archives of Disease in Childhood*, 88, 53-6

Jones, J M, Lawson, M L, Daneman, D, Olmsted, M P and Rodin, G (2000) Eating disorders in adolescent females with and without type 1 diabetes: cross sectional study, *British Medical Journal*, 320, 1563-6

Jones, M E, Swerdlow, A J, Gill, L E and Goldacre, M J (1998) Pre-natal and early life risk factors for childhood onset diabetes mellitus: a record linkage study, *International Journal of Epidemiology*, 27, 444-9

Kaufman, F R (2002) Type 2 diabetes in children and young adults: a 'new epidemic', *Clinical Diabetes*, 20, 217-18

Kipps, S, Bahu, T, Ong, K, Ackland, F M, Brown, R S, Fox, C T, Griffin, N K, Knight, A H, Mann, N P, Neil, H A W, Simpson, H , Edge, J A and Dunger, D B (2002) Current methods of transfer of young people with type 1 diabetes to adult services, *Diabetic Medicine*, 19, 8, 649-54

Kovacs, M, Goldston, D, Obrosky, D and Bonar, L K (1997a) Psychiatric disorders in youths with IDDM: rates and risk factors, *Diabetes Care*, 20, 1, 36-44

Kovacs, M, Obrosky, D, Goldston, D and Drash, A (1997b) Major depressive disorder in youths with IDDM: controlled prospective study of course and outcome, *Diabetes Care*, 20, 1, 45-51

Kurtz, Z, Mawer, C and Hopkins, A 'Guidelines for the transfer of young people with chronic physical disorders from paediatric to adult services' *in* Kurtz, Z and Hopkins, A *eds* (1996) *Services for young people with chronic disorders in their transition from childhood to adult life*. Royal College of Physicians

La Greca, A M, Swales, T, Klemp, S, Madigan, S and Skyler, J (1995a) Adolescents with diabetes: gender differences in psychosocial functioning and glycaemic control, *Children's Health Care*, 24, 1, 61-78

La Greca, A M, Auslander, W F, Greco, P, Spetter, D, Fisher, E B Jr. and Santiago, J V (1995b) I get by with a little help from my family and friends: support for diabetes care, *Journal of Pediatric Psychology*, 20, 4, 449-76

Lightfoot, J Mukherjee, S and Sloper, P (2001) Supporting pupils with special health needs in mainstream schools: policy and practice, *Children & Society*, 15, 57-69

Lustman, P J, Griffith, L S, Gavard, J A and Cloue, R E (1992) Depression in adults with diabetes, *Diabetes Care*, 15, 11, 1631-9

McKinney, P A, Okasha, M, Parslow, R C, Law, G R, Gurney, K A, Williams, R and Bodansky, H J (2000) Early social mixing and childhood type 1 diabetes mellitus: a case-control study in Yorkshire, UK, *Diabetes Medicine*, 17, 3, 236-42

Marteau, T M, Bloch, S and Baum, J D (1987) Family life and diabetic control, *Journal of Child Psychology and Psychiatry*, 28, 6 823-33

Meltzer, L J, Bennett Johnson, S, Prine, J M, Banks, R A, Desrosiers, P M and Silverstein, J H (2001) Disordered eating, body mass, and glycaemic control in adolescents with type 1 diabetes, *Diabetes Care*, 24, 678-82

Miller-Johnson, S, Emery, R E, Marvin, R, Clarke, W, Lovinger, R and Martin, M (1994) Parent–child relationships and the management of insulin-dependent diabetes mellitus, *Journal of Consulting and Clinical Psychology*, 62, 3, 603-10

Morris, A D, Boyle, D I R, McMahon, A D, Greene, S A, MacDonald, T M and Newton, R W for the DARTS/MEMO Collaboration (1997) Adherence to insulin treatment, glycaemic control, and ketoacidosis in insulin-dependent diabetes mellitus, *The Lancet*, 350, 9090,1505-10

Mukherjee, S, Lightfoot, J and Sloper, P (2000) *Improving communication between health and education for children with chronic illness or physical disability* York: University of York

Mukherjee, S, Lightfoot, J and Sloper, P (2002) Communicating about pupils in mainstream school with special health needs: the NHS perspective, *Child Care, Health & Development*, 28, 1, 21-7

Neumark-Sztainer, D, Patterson, J, Mellin, A, Ackard, D M, Utter, J, Story, M and Sockalosky, J (2002) Weight control practices and disordered eating behaviours among adolescent females and males with type 1 diabetes, *Diabetes Care*, 25, 8, 1289-96

Newnham, A, Ryan, R and Khunti, K (2002) Prevalence of diagnosed diabetes mellitus in general practice in England and Wales, 1994 to 1998, *Health Statistics Quarterly*, 14, Summer

NHS Scotland (2001) *Scottish Diabetes Framework*. Scottish Executive

Nissim, R, Rodin, G, Daneman, D, Rydall, A, Colton, P, Maharaj, S and Jones, J (2002) Eating disturbances in adolescent girls with type 1 diabetes mellitus, *Harefuah*, 141, 10, 902-7

Ó Dochartaigh, N (2002) *The internet research handbook: a practical guide for students and researchers in the social sciences.* Sage

Olsen, R and Sutton, J (1998) More hassle, more alone: adolescents with diabetes and the role of formal and informal support, *Child: Care, Health and Development*, 24, 1, 31-9

Parslow, R C, McKinney, P A, Law, G R and Bodansky, H J (2001) Population mixing and childhood diabetes, *International Journal of Epidemiology*, 30, 3, 533-8

Peveler, R C, Fairburn, C G, Boller, I and Dunger, D (1992) Eating disorders in adolescents with IDDM. A controlled study, *Diabetes Care*, 15, 10, 1356-60

Pita, R, Fotakopoulou, O, Kiosseoglou, G, Zafiri, M, Roikou, K, Simos, G, Didaggelos, T and Karamitsos, D (2002) Depression, quality of life and diabetes mellitus, *Hippokratia*, 6, Supplement 1

Rangasami, J J, Greenwood, D C, McSporran, B, Smail, P J, Patterson, C C and Waugh, N R on behalf of the Scottish Study Group for the Care of Young Diabetics (1997) Rising incidence of type 1 diabetes in Scottish children 1984–93, *Archives of Disease in Childhood*, 77, 210–3

Sawyer, S M, Zalan, A and Bond, L M (2002) Telephone reminders improve adolescent clinic attendance: randomised control trial, *Journal of Paediatrics and Child Health*, 38, 1, 79-83

Scottish Executive (2001) *Scottish Diabetes Framework*. Scottish Executive

Shepherd, M, Sparkes, A C and Hattersley, A T (2001) Genetic testing in maturity onset diabetes of the young, *Practical Diabetes International*, 18, 1, 16-21

Shiell, A W, Campbell, D M, Hall, M H and Barker, D J (2000) Diet in late pregnancy and glucose-insulin metabolism of the offspring 40 years later, *British Journal of Obstetrics and Gynaecology*, 107, 7, 890-5

SIGN (2001) *Management of diabetes*. Scottish Intercollegiate Guidelines Network (SIGN Publication No. 55)

Simmons, A V, Atkinson, K, Atkinson, P and Cross, B (1997) Failure of patients to attend a medical outpatient clinic, *Journal of the Royal College of Physicians of London*, 31, 1, 70-3

Skinner, T C and Hampson, S E (1998) Social support and personal models of diabetes in relation to self-care and well-being in adolescents with type 1 diabetes mellitus, *Journal of Adolescence*, 21, 703-15

Smith, A H K (2001) *The National Paediatric Diabetes Audit: Annual Report 2001*. Diabetes UK

Stene, L C, Hongve, H, Magnus, P, Rønningen, K S and Joner, G (2002) Acidic drinking water and risk of childhood-onset type 1 diabetes, *Diabetes Care*, 25, 1534-8

Stene, L C, Magnus, P, Lie, R T, Oddmund, S, Joner, G and the Norwegian Childhood Diabetes Study Group (2001) Birth weight and childhood onset type 1 diabetes: population based cohort study, *British Medical Journal*, 322, 889-92

Stobbs, P (2001) *Special Educational Needs and Disability Act 2001: Schools' duties in the Disability Discrimination Act 1995*. National Children's Bureau

Tatman, M A and Lessing, D N (1993) Can we improve diabetes care in schools?, *Archives of Disease in Childhood*, 69, 4, 450-1

Turner, B (1998) The growing problem of diabetes, *Times Health Supplement*, April, 6-7

Turner, J and Kelly, B (2000) Emotional dimensions of chronic illness, *Western Journal of Medicine*, 172, 124-8

Viner, R (1999) Transition from paediatric to adult care. Bridging the gaps or passing the buck?, *Archives of Disease in Childhood*, 81, 3, 271-5

Viner, R, McGrath, M and Trudinger, P (1996) Family stress and metabolic control in diabetes, *Archives of Disease in Childhood*, 74, 418-21

Watson, M and Forshaw, M (2002) Child outpatient non-attendance may indicate welfare concerns, *British Medical Journal*, 324, 739

Weissberg-Benchell, J, Glasgow, A M, Tynan, W D, Wirtz, P, Turek, J and Ward, J (1995) Adolescent diabetes management and mismanagement, *Diabetes Care*, 18, 1, 77-82

Wilson, R J, Christie, M J and Bradley, C (1998) A qualitative investigation to inform the design of quality of life measures for children with diabetes, *Diabetic Medicine*, 15, S46

Wilson, S J and Greenhalgh, S (1999) Keeping in touch with young people – where have all the DNA'ers gone?, *Practical Diabetes*, 16, 3, 87-8

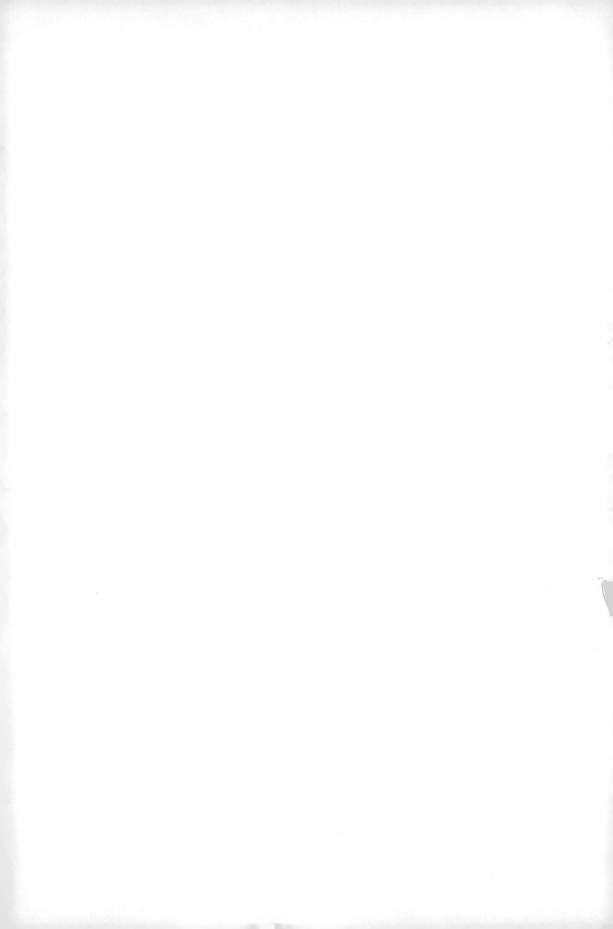